EMBARKS NURSING ON A ROAD THAT NEEDS TO BE TAKEN...

"From a philosophical and nursing process perspective, this innovative manual outlines approaches, techniques, and strategies for nursing practice via the telephone. Practitioners, students, and nurse educators will find this manual useful in all practice and teaching/learning environments."

—Loretta C. Ford, RN, EdD, FAAN
Professor and Dean Emeritus
University of Rochester School of Nursing
Rochester, New York

"*Telephone Nursing: The Process* embarks nursing on a road that needs to be taken...beyond the bedside, curative approach to care into the challenge of prevention and interaction with the ambulatory client."

—Mary Jo Gilmer, RN, MSN, MBA
Assistant Clinical Professor
Queens College
Charlotte Memorial Hospital and Medical Center
Charlotte, North Carolina

"An extraordinary workbook. Every nurse who interacts with the ambulatory public should have a copy. It guides the nurse, in outline format, through the nursing process as it can occur over the telephone (and, incidentally, gives a wide variety of examples of interviewing techniques which are also useful eye-to-eye). It relates problems identified over the phone to nursing diagnoses and functional health patterns and suggests interventions appropriate to the telephone. It also includes course objectives, worksheet, and tools for a telephone nurse training program."

—Colleen Conway-Welch
Professor and Dean
Vanderbilt University
Nashville, Tennessee

To Tom!
With love and thanks!
Sandy

November 1, 1990

INVALUABLE...PRACTICAL...CREATIVE...

"This manual is a 'must' for every emergency or outpatient department nurse, manager, clinical specialist or nurse practitioner. A practical, straightforward, holistic approach to developing, implementing, and evaluating a telephone nursing system. Excellent as an interactive tool for staff education."

—James J. Hoelz, RN, MS, FNPC, CEN
Nurse Manager/Emergency Department
Mercer Medical Center
Trenton, New Jersey

"Ambulatory care administrators responsible for staff resource allocation will find this text invaluable in utilizing staff efficiently and in reaching untapped markets. Risk management is addressed by approach and through use of physician-approved guidelines. A creative, cost-effective enhancement to physician practices, hospitals, and other healthcare providers."

—Peggy Sawyer, RN, MSN, CS, MBA
Manager/Hospital Operations Consulting
Ernst & Young
New York, New York

"*Telephone Nursing: The Process* is an exercise in entrepreneurial practice. The authors are to be congratulated for not only identifying a need and responding to it, but assuring that professional cognitive skills are practiced and presented to the public. This can only enhance the image of the professional nurse as well as provide a needed service."

—Roxane Spitzer-Lehmann, RN, FAAN, MA, MBA
Corporate Vice President
St. Joseph Health System
Orange, California

"The content was quite thorough and complete. The break-out sections (i.e., communication skills, personnel selection) were particularly helpful and insightful from my point of view, plus being easy to read and flowing well. As health care continues to change focusing more on 'empowering' patients to become involved and responsible for their healthcare concerns, nursing triage will serve as a primary education tool in making that happen. This book is a valuable resource for nursing as telephone triaging systems become increasingly important."

—E. Mary Johnson, RN, BSN
Director, Outpatient Clinic Nursing
Cleveland Clinic
Cleveland, Ohio

NEW AND EXCITING...
A MUST-READ FOR NURSING LEADERS AND VISIONARIES...

"In an age when information, resource allocation, and utilization affect the in-patient institution, this book offers fresh, new methods for gaining market edge. This text puts nursing process at the very edge of revenue production with special attention to client relationships that so often determine choice of healthcare provider. A must-read for nursing leaders and visionaries. A book that is right on time."

—Robert E. Blake, MS, RN, CNS
Assistant Director of Nursing
Texas Children's Hospital
Houston, Texas

"*Telephone Nursing: The Process* provides nurses with a new approach to the nursing process. Technological advances demand that nurses be skilled in interviewing techniques as well as finding solutions for problems even when they cannot see or feel the patient. This book brings it all together and provides a basis from which to start the process."

—Janet L. Snow, RN, DNSc
President
National Health Systems, Inc.
Burr Ridge, Illinois

"A new and exciting alternative for the healthcare consumer..."

—Rebecca Cherry Kreppner, RN, MBA, PhD
Assistant Professor
Texas Woman's University
Houston, Texas

"I have reviewed this book rather thoroughly and find it an outstanding review of what nursing by telephone requires. The placement of this nursing function within the overall nursing process is especially important because of the level of professional expertise necessary to fill this role safely and realistically. It occurs to me that the book will fill an important need not only for nurses but for physicians and administrators as well. The clarity outlined regarding the nursing process as opposed to providing medical advice should be especially reassuring to our medical and management colleagues. The authors have done an outstanding job of differentiating the practices."

—Sarah S. Detmer, MSN
Director of Nursing Services and
Assistant Dean, School of Nursing
Medical College of Virginia Hospitals
Richmond, Virginia

TAKES NURSING TO NEW HEIGHTS...

"The authors have masterfully shared their collective wealth of experience in a well-written and well-designed presentation. This book is an extraordinarily practical learning tool and reference for nurses involved with increasingly important telecommunications mechanisms of providing health care services. The book is user friendly, covers key points, and is appropriate for various levels of nursing students, staff, and other ambulatory care personnel."

—Violet H. Barkauskas, PhD, RN, FAAN
Associate Dean for Administration
Associate Professor, Community Health Nursing
University of Michigan School of Nursing
Ann Arbor, Michigan

"We find this to be an *excellent*, well-organized book based upon sound experience, philosophy, and principles. It will be very useful in our ambulatory settings where nurses must frequently practice telephone nursing with our established patients."

—Doris M. Armstrong, MEd, RN, FAAN
Vice President for Nursing
—Joyce E. Schickler, RNC, MS
Director of Nursing, Emergency Center
Ambulatory & Psychiatric Services, Hartford Hospital
Hartford, Connecticut

"This book is a long overdue guide for the registered nurse who must assess a caller objectively without the benefit of seeing him or her. It provides a structured format for defining the role, responsibilities, and implications of telephone nursing while assuring that the caller will receive consistent, appropriate advice. This information is a 'must' in establishing a telephone nursing role in *any* organization."

—Carolyn C. Boyle, RN, MBA
Senior Manager
Ernst & Young

"*Telephone Nursing: The Process* takes nursing to new heights. The challenge to deliver comprehensive care in a consumer-driven market, while balancing costs, requires a very creative approach. The expansion of nursing-care delivery via the telephone meets that challenge. Administrators, nurse managers, physicians, and direct-care providers will find this operationalized concept to be a realistic and very avant-garde way to approach today's pressing delivery concerns."

—Julee T. Marker, RN, MSN, CPQA
Director/Critical Care
Baptist Medical Center of Oklahoma
Oklahoma City, Oklahoma

TELEPHONE NURSING: THE PROCESS

TRIAGE, HEALTH INFORMATION, RESOURCES, AND REFERRAL

SANDRA MATHERLY, RNC, FNP, MA
SHANNON HODGES, MBA

CONTRIBUTORS
Thomas W. Filardo, MD
Dianne Maxwell, RNC, MSN

Center for Research in Ambulatory Health Care Administration
Denver, Colorado

Printed in the United States of America.

International Standard Book Number: 0-933948-23-9

For the nurses who practice on the phone and the patients they serve.

Telephone nurses are highly skilled, creative problem solvers who are committed to providing high-quality care including triage, case finding, health information, and referrals. These merit special mention:

> The NURSE ON CALL Nurses at St. Mary's Medical Center, Knoxville, Tennessee
>
> The Patient Referral Nurses, Telephone Advice Nurses, and Family Practice-Mahomet Nurses at the Carle Clinic, Urbana, Illinois
>
> The Dial-A-Nurse Nurses at the McKinley Health Center, University of Illinois, Urbana, Illinois

ABOUT THE AUTHORS

Sandra Matherly, RNC, FNP, MA, is a principal of a consulting group specializing in ambulatory care with a focus on telephone nursing. Nurse on Call®, the firm's turn-key telephone nursing program, includes specialized telephone nursing education and training, and operations and marketing consulting to create telephone nursing programs customized to the client organization's needs.

Ms. Matherly has been involved with telephone nursing for the last six years. At Carle Clinic in Urbana, Illinois, she had responsibility for revising and expanding telephone nursing services. After leaving her management position at Carle and finishing her graduate management education, she became involved with telephone nursing programs across the country implemented by a variety of organizations: health maintenance organizations, medical centers, hospital emergency rooms, and university health services.

With over twenty years of nursing and nursing management experience, Ms. Matherly has achieved visibility in her field through publishing, public speaking, educational endeavors, and professional affiliations. In recognition of exceptional skills, abilities, and excellence in practice and management, she received a national award and was designated a Commonwealth Fund Nurse Executive Scholar.

Ms. Matherly is a certified nurse practitioner with extensive ambulatory care experience: seven years spent in emergency department nursing and supervision, and fifteen years in a large multispecialty group practice and a small family practice satellite clinic. Her academic appointments include schools of nursing (where she taught ambulatory care nursing) and the University of Illinois College of Medicine. Her academic credentials include a diploma from the Johns Hopkins School of Nursing, a bachelor of science degree in nursing from the University of Illinois at Chicago, and a master of arts degree in human resource management from the University of Illinois at Urbana-Champaign, Institute of Labor and Industrial Relations.

Shannon Hodges, MBA, also a principal of the firm, is the marketing and communications director for Nurse on Call. Ms. Hodges has an extensive background in healthcare and medical marketing and communications, having had primary responsibility for the creation of publications and marketing materials aimed at physicians, nurses, and other healthcare professionals. She is an experienced writer and researcher, and has acted as a consultant to medical device and healthcare organizations since 1985.

Ms. Hodges has planned and implemented training programs and seminars for students, management professionals, and nurses on a variety of topics. Her academic credentials include a bachelor of science degree in organizational development from the University of California, Davis, and a master of business administration degree in marketing from the University of Illinois at Urbana-Champaign.

CONTENTS

List of Figures xiv
Preface xv

CHAPTER ONE
WHAT IS TELEPHONE NURSING? 1

The Right Thing at the Right Time 3
A Vital Link in the Healthcare System 5
The Nurse on Call® Approach 6
Goals, Concepts, Definitions 8
A Call for New Levels of Expertise 10
Roles and Responsibilities 12
Special Problems 15

CHAPTER TWO
THE TELEPHONE NURSING PROCESS 17

Assessment 20
Interviewing 20
Listening 21
Assessing Symptoms 22
Considering the Holistic View 23
Problem Definition 24
The Problem-Oriented Approach 25
The Nursing Diagnosis Approach 29
Planning 32
Implementation 32
Evaluation 32

CHAPTER THREE
THE ART OF COMMUNICATING 33

Words + Emotion = Message 35
Establishing Trustworthiness 36
Active Listening 37
Dealing with Emotions 39
The Difficult Caller 41
Patient Persuasion and Education 43

CHAPTER FOUR
SPECIAL PATIENT POPULATIONS 49

Infants and Children 51
Adolescents 52
Young Adults 53
Women 54
Men 63
Seniors 64
Cultural Issues 68

CHAPTER FIVE
TAKING THE TELEPHONE HISTORY 71

Chief Complaint 73
Present Illness 75
Past History 76
Review of Systems 76

CHAPTER SIX
PERSONNEL CONSIDERATIONS 81

Position Requirements 83
Standards and Performance Criteria 84
Clinical Practice 84
Education 86
Leadership 87
Professionalism 88
Job Description 89

CHAPTER SEVEN
PUTTING IT ALL TOGETHER 93

Documentation 97
Practice Standards 97
Legal Issues 99
Guidelines for Practice 100

Appendix A. American Nurses' Association Code for Nurses 107

Appendix B. International Council of Nurses Code for Nurses 111

Appendix C. Nurse on Call® Telephone Nursing Training Program Course Objectives 113

Appendix D. Telephone Nursing Program Sample Documentation Form 115

Appendix E. Nursing Assessment Worksheet and Tools 117

Appendix F. Peer Evaluation Form 121

Appendix G. Discussion Exercises 123

Appendix H. The Nurse on Call® Program 125

References 127

LIST OF FIGURES

1. Patient Resources 6
2. Patient "Balance Sheet" 7
3. Required Areas of Expertise for the Telephone Nurse 12
4. Roles and Responsibilities of the Telephone Nurse 13
5. The Nursing Process: In-Person v. Via Telephone 14
6. The Nursing Process Cycle 19
7. Symptom Assessment 25
8. Classes of Patient Problems 26
9. Become a Better Solution Generator 28
10. Differences Between Medical Diagnosis and Nursing Diagnosis 30
11. Nursing Diagnoses Common to Ambulatory Care Settings 31
12. Useful Synonyms for Telephone Nursing 38
13. Active Listening Skills 40
14. Understanding Beliefs, Attitudes, and Values Behind Patient Behaviors 45
15. Continuum of Patient Descriptors 47
16. Women's Health-Related Roles 59
17. Telephone Nursing Quick Assessment Process 96
18. Important Resources 98
19. Most Frequent Allegations Against Nurses and Prevention Tips 101

PREFACE

The telephone has long been a difficult area to all working in ambulatory care: receptionists, technicians, nurses, and physicians. There are special problems inherent in giving advice via the telephone that is appropriate for time, place, and provider — whether the advice is for triage, case finding, resource identification, or referral.

This book was written to provide a planned approach to telephone nursing. It is based on the nursing process, a systematic method of decision making and problem solving, and the orientation is holistic, primary nursing, and case finding.

We offer an overview of the areas where we believe nursing skills must exceed the norm in order to deliver high-quality telephone nursing. Also discussed are the organizational considerations that our experiences have proven to be essential in the creation of an organized telephone nursing program.

This information should be useful to nurses and others working in the diverse ambulatory care settings, including group practices, hospital emergency departments and outpatient areas, community health programs, and physician offices. It should also be helpful to students of ambulatory care, receptionists, and technicians.

Our intent is to improve the efficiency and effectiveness of telephone nursing care, to stimulate professional growth, and ultimately to benefit all ambulatory care professionals, organizations, and the patients whom we serve.

We wish to acknowledge many people for their contributions to this work. These contributions took a variety of forms, including writing portions of a chapter, collecting needed information, providing technical assistance, reviewing concepts or text, and providing support and encouragement.

Jane Dailey, Vice President/Patient Care Services, St. Mary's Medical Center, Knoxville, Tennessee, whose vision, support, and expertise were with us from the beginning and helped this book become a reality

Thomas Filardo, MD, and Dianne Maxwell, RNC, MSN, who reviewed the text from medical, nurse practitioner, and educator perspectives, and contributed to the "Review of Systems" chapter

Melvin Ehrhardt, MD, JD, who reviewed the text from medical and legal perspectives

Carolyn Boyle, RN, MBA, Senior Manager, Ernst & Young, Walnut Creek, California, who carefully reviewed and made suggestions regarding the qualifications, roles and responsibilities of nurses

James B. Corbett, MD, who provided assistance in the area of pediatrics

Ruth Inman, RN; DiAnne Haines, RN; and Sally Roth, RN; who served as professional nursing role models

Linda Johnson, RN, HMO Health Services Director, who assisted from the perspective of nursing in an HMO model

Sandra Reifsteck, RN, MS, FACMGA, Associate Administrator, Carle Clinic, Urbana, Illinois, who played a major role in initiating telephone nursing in the Carle organization and who has lent her support and encouragement to the writing of this book

Linda D'Angelo, MSN, MBA, Patient Care Director, Carle Clinic, and the assistant directors who provided their thoughtful review and suggestions

Tamara Mitchell, MD, Family Practice Department Head and Telephone Advice Medical Advisor/Director, Carle Clinic, who offered her review, support and encouragement

Jack Pollard, MD; Roger Powell, MD; and Bob Parker, MD, physician executives at Carle who supported the development and expansion of telephone nursing services

The physicians and staff of Carle-Mahomet who gave us their support

Karen Knutson, MSN, MBA, Former Nursing Director, McKinley Health Service, University of Illinois, who lent us her support and reviewed one of the earliest versions of this work

Burt Waller, Executive Vice President, St Mary's Medical Center, Knoxville, Tennessee, who supported the development of hospital-based Nurse on Call

Dale Brown, MSN, Project Director; Gay Harrison, ER Nursing Manager; and Vivian James, RN, Nursing Manager, at St. Mary's Nurse on Call Telephone Nursing Program, who made suggestions from the perspective of hospital-based telephone nursing

Lynn Massingale, MD, Southeastern Emergency Physicians, Knoxville, Tennessee, who provided information regarding hospital-based telephone nursing in eastern Tennessee

Ann Cavanaugh, RN, Director of Nursing, The Springfield Clinic, Springfield, Illinois, and Springfield area nurses who provided information concerning the needs of ambulatory nurses in diverse settings

Sharon Strack, RN, Nursing Manager, Level I Trauma Center and Emergency Department, Carle Foundation Hospital, Urbana, Illinois, who provided information concerning the issues of telephone nursing in emergency departments

Daniel Gregorie, MD, President, ChoiceCare, Cincinnati, Ohio, and former physician executive at New England Kaiser, who provided information and support concerning telephone nursing as a positive, cost-effective physician support service and marketing advantage

The nurses, physicians, and staff of the Palo Alto Medical Foundation, Palo Alto, California, who provided information concerning issues and needs from a group practice perspective

Joyce Schickler, Director of Nursing for Ambulatory Care, Flight Nursing and Psychiatry, Hartford Hospital, Hartford, Connecticut, who provided valuable information about ambulatory care nursing issues and approaches in a large, urban medical center

Lynda Nauright, PhD, Assistant Dean, Emory University School of Nursing, Atlanta, Georgia, who provided support and information about nursing student needs

Mary Jane Donough, RN, and Mary Farr, NP, former nursing instructors, The Johns Hopkins School of Nursing; Ingeborg Mauksch, RN, PhD, Sanibel Island, Florida; and Loretta Ford, RN, EdD, Rochester, New York; who were Sandy's mentors and so very important in developing her professional nursing philosophy, commitment, and leadership

The Commonwealth Fund of New York, New York, who continues to support professional nursing and the development and education of nursing leaders

Peggy Greene, Janice Pramik, and staff members at the Center for Research in Ambulatory Health Care Administration (CRAHCA), Denver, Colorado, who provided their invaluable assistance in publishing this work

Last but not least, we wish to thank our friends and family, especially our husbands, Joe and Bob.

CHAPTER ONE

WHAT IS TELEPHONE NURSING?

It's zooming to the top of the charts. Telephone nursing is one of the fastest growing areas of nursing specialization. Almost every nurse practicing in ambulatory care today engages in some form of telephone nursing for some percentage of the time. The growth in this area reflects the dramatic demographic, social, and economic changes that have occurred in the last twenty years in the United States healthcare system. The evolving healthcare needs of the American people and the transformation of the structure of healthcare reimbursement and delivery systems have created the need for highly skilled, specially trained telephone nurses and organized telephone nursing systems.

THE RIGHT THING AT THE RIGHT TIME

Telephone nursing, in centralized and decentralized configurations, offers answers to some of the biggest challenges facing providers today in their attempts to provide high-quality, cost-effective care. Telephone nursing:

- decreases the wasteful use of emergency settings for non-emergency care
- increases the accessibility of the healthcare system to all patients, regardless of their ability to pay or their familiarity with medical procedures, systems, and practitioners
- increases patient satisfaction, especially with after-hours care
- matches patients with appropriate physicians and services

Telephone nursing is the "right thing at the right time." For many problems faced by today's healthcare organizations, clinicians and their patients, telephone nursing services offer a set of solutions.

DIVERSE CONSUMER NEEDS. Today's healthcare consumers are, in many ways, a study in extremes. On one end of the continuum are those who are seeking more and more information in order to make decisions regarding their own health care. They choose which physicians to see and which hospitals and clinics to utilize, and they actively seek out healthcare educational opportunities. These consumers benefit greatly from telephone nursing because it provides them with the quick answers they seek from their providers.

At the opposite end of the continuum are those who are on the "outside" of the healthcare system: the underinsured and the uninsured. The care-seeking behavior of these consumers is focused on obtaining care only when a problem becomes an emergency. Telephone nursing is an important service for these populations as well as for the active information-seekers. The underinsured and the uninsured have an acute need for easy access to healthcare information and referral since they have little regular contact with healthcare professionals.

OVERCROWDED EMERGENCY ROOMS. Through its triaging function, telephone nursing can help to ease the inappropriate use of emergency rooms (ERs). Many emergency rooms are not only facing greater numbers of emergency patients (as more and more ERs close their doors), but they also must cope with the swelling number of non-emergency patients who lack a primary-care physician. Some of these patients can be referred to appropriate, non-emergency care. The patient, too, will benefit by avoiding the long waiting time faced by non-emergency ER patients. Telephone nursing, in this scenario, not only makes efficient use of resources, but also increases patient satisfaction with access to care.

RESOURCE AND LIABILITY MANAGEMENT. Telephone nursing is a function of all ambulatory-care nurses at one time or another. The amount of time nurses spend on the phone has increased in recent years, to the point where it now makes up a significant portion of many nurses' duties. Without an organized telephone nursing service, however, many nurses may have no formalized nursing guidelines from which to make assessments, no approved procedures to follow, no standardized means of documenting calls, no structured education or training specifically for nursing via the phone, no quality assurance process. In short, they have no means of providing consistent, high-quality care for their patients and no means of protecting themselves and their employers from the risks inherent in telephone nursing.

The ER nurse is frequently asked to speak to patients on the phone about their health concerns. These calls often simply pull the nurse away from his or her "true" job, which is the care of patients in the ER in need of emergency care. Because these nurses are often not operating under specific guidelines and policies, most will take the safest route and ask the patient to come to the ER. This practice leads to increased costs and the waste of valuable resources — the specialist talents in the ER. It also contributes to overcrowding and leads to consumer frustration and dissatisfaction. An organized telephone nursing service, with nurses specifically chosen and educated to practice telephone nursing, eliminates the problem of ER nurses being "pulled away" from their primary duties.

A VITAL LINK IN THE HEALTHCARE SYSTEM

Although the focus here is on telephone nursing, the foundations of this book lie in the person-to-person and clinical skills gained through education and practice. This philosophy of telephone nursing is based on a strong commitment to whole-person nursing care — care which recognizes the unique assets each patient brings to maintaining and regaining health. The concepts and approach are focused on the telephone nurse, but they are appropriate for all ambulatory care.

To provide successful nursing care via the telephone, a nurse needs to have strong ambulatory-care nursing skills as well as a commitment to responsibility and service. Good telephone nurses are dedicated to providing individualized care. One of their most important functions is to help make the bureaucracy and technology of modern medicine understandable to patients by explaining services, medications, procedures, health conditions, and specialized medical jargon in human terms, appropriate for the patient's level of education and experience. This information is dispensed by the nurse with compassion and caring to help ease the patient's anxiety.

Telephone nurses improve access to care by identifying available services and resources. As both guide and interpreter within the healthcare maze, they lower financial and informational barriers, allowing consumers to make informed decisions. They provide education to assist individuals and families in developing a broad range of health-promoting behaviors. They encourage self-care by teaching techniques for health maintenance and illness prevention. They are in a position to "sell" self-care and to follow through with the medical regimen, which simultaneously serves the needs of patients, physicians, and an overburdened healthcare system.

Healthcare consumers are asking more questions which the telephone nurse is fortunately in a position to answer. Patients who want to assume more responsibility for their own health care can be helped in this effort by telephone nurses. Telephone contact can provide them with information and can assist them in creating strategies for health. Telephone nursing practice includes preventive-care activities which produce cost advantages by averting more complicated, costly care further down the road. Through effective teaching and information sharing, telephone nurses help patients to engage in appropriate health behaviors or, if sick, to regain health.

Preventive-care activities are appropriate in all ambulatory-care settings and with all patient populations, in primary care as well as subspecialty

FIGURE 1. PATIENT RESOURCES

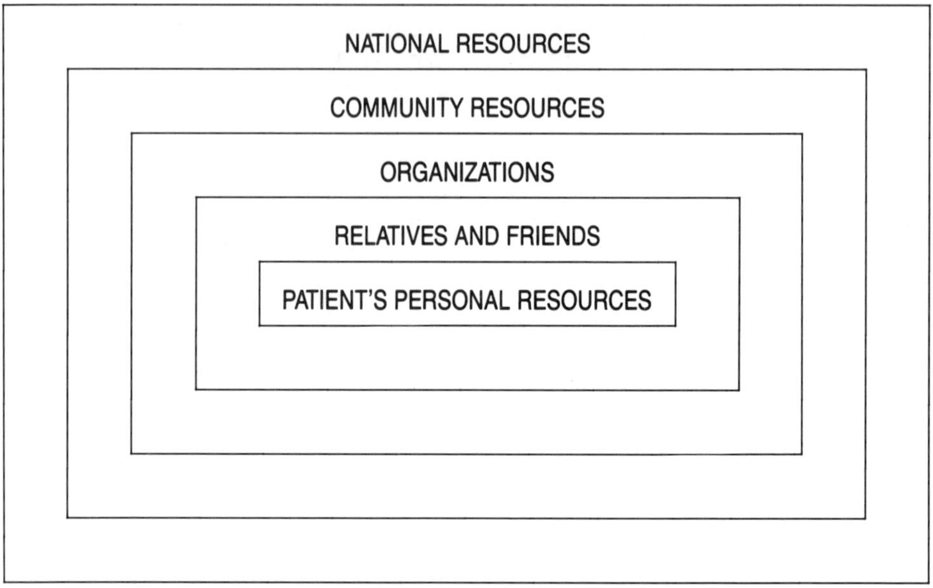

areas. The approach stays the same: the telephone nurse, working with the physician responsible for the patient's medical care, provides the best possible nursing care — triage, case finding, access to the healthcare system, information, liaison functions, resource identification, and referrals.

In essence, telephone nurses comprise a vital link between the healthcare needs of people and the complex, and often confusing, system through which healthcare services are provided.

THE NURSE ON CALL® APPROACH

Patients are complex individuals, each of whom brings different "assets and liabilities" to their efforts to gain, regain, or maintain health. In 1898 in *Notes on Nursing*, Florence Nightingale wrote, "The nurse nurses the sick, not the sickness." It is this basic nursing philosophy — holistic and case finding — that underlies the Nurse on Call philosophy of telephone nursing.

A caller may ask, "What are the symptoms of drug abuse?" The skilled nurse will then ask herself, "What are the needs of this person? What is the real reason for this call? Is the person concerned about himself? Is there someone else in this person's life who is abusing drugs?" It is the

FIGURE 2. PATIENT "BALANCE SHEET"

ASSETS	LIABILITIES
PERSONAL • PSYCHOLOGICAL • PHYSICAL • FINANCIAL FAMILIAL FRIENDS COMMUNITY CULTURAL	ACUTE AND CHRONIC DISORDERS • PSYCHOLOGICAL • PHYSICAL RESOURCE DEFICITS SOCIAL PROBLEMS

responsibility of the nurse to assess patient needs and to respond appropriately with information, resource identification, and referral, rather than a simple answer to the question.

The Nurse on Call approach is based on consideration of patient risk factors, such as age, sex, present and past health history, and psychosocial factors (socioeconomic and cultural issues, for example). It requires a sensitivity to the influence of physical, psychological, and social environments on the individual and his or her family. These influences require expertise in nursing assessment and intervention, including the ability to employ all steps of the nursing process with success.

The telephone nurse must have strong skills in the following areas: communication, thorough assessment, structured history taking, creative problem solving, and accurate documentation. All steps of the nursing process — assessment, diagnosis, plan implementation, and evaluation — are used by the effective telephone nurse to create an accurate picture of the patient's problems and available resources (see *Figure 1*). An evaluation of the patient's "balance sheet" of "assets and liabilities" can be helpful (see *Figure 2*). The liabilities are those very problems which the caller is now experiencing, as well as those factors that led to the problems. The assets are those factors which will help the caller to solve those problems.

The telephone nurse must be skilled in recognizing the appropriate scope of nursing practice over the phone. The nurse must be able to determine when a physician needs to be consulted, and whether activities are medically dependent or independent in nature. Not only must the appropriate level of practice be identified, but it must be articulated as well. Appropriate nursing practice should be clearly defined so that it does not inadvertently become the practice of medicine over the phone. This is critical to providing the best care at the least risk to the organization and the nurse.

GOALS, CONCEPTS, DEFINITIONS

What is nursing? Finding the answer to this question is not a simple task. Indeed, there are a number of nursing theorists who have devoted much of their professional lives to defining and, therefore, directing nursing practice and education.

To achieve a goal, everybody involved must clearly articulate the goal, and then decide how they will attempt to achieve the goal. Nursing has been hampered by unclear or overly ambitious goals that were not measurable. Most theorists do agree that nursing has something to do with health, but health is also not so easily defined. In the past, health was defined simply as "the absence of disease." Then, the World Health Organization's definition of health was created: "complete mental, physical, social, and spiritual well-being." The problem with such an ambitious definition is, first, no one can achieve it, and second, no one can measure how close one is toward its achievement (for example, is the patient 80 percent healthy yet?).

A newer, less ambitious model for health has been developed by Mary Josephine Flaherty, PhD, RN. This model provides realistic goals, and is both attainable and measurable:

> "...health is a measure of the competence with which individuals and families function in their environments. Thus, an individual's health state is a measure of functional competence" (Curtin 1984, p.8).

A reasonable definition of nursing, given this definition of health, is:

> "Nursing is helping people attain, retain, or regain health" (Schlotfeldt 1972, p.245-6).

The following operational definitions and concepts are provided to clarify the outlook represented in this book.

HEALTH. Health is a measure of the competence with which individuals and families function in their environments (Curtin 1984).

NURSING. Nursing is helping people to attain, retain, or regain health, and being accountable for the quality of that care (Schlotfeldt 1972).

PATIENT. The patient is the individual experiencing the problem or concern precipitating the call. Although the terms "caller" and "patient" are used interchangeably throughout this book, it should be recognized that at times, the caller will be the patient's parent, spouse, adult child, or friend.

PRIMARY NURSING. The primary nurse provides individualized, holistic care to the patient. The primary nurse makes a professional commitment to direct and ensure comprehensive care to the patient, and is accountable for the quality of that care. He or she collaborates with other healthcare professionals to provide the best possible care for the patient and acts as the patient's advocate within the healthcare system. Primary nursing makes the broad concept of professional commitment to patients and their families a functional reality (Zander 1980). The Nurse on Call nurse bases her professional practice on the philosophy of primary nursing.

TELEPHONE NURSING GUIDELINES. The guidelines upon which this book is based are physician approved and organizationally sanctioned guidelines for patient assessment, triaging, and referral. They assist the nurse in the assessment, problem definition, and planning phases of the call. These guidelines are designed to maximize the level of information and assistance given to the caller, while minimizing the risk to the organization and the nurse.

STAFFING CONCERNS. Telephone nursing is truly expanded nursing care involving clinical decisions. It is impossible to predict the nature of calls, and decisions often must be made based on the expertise of a professional nurse who identifies and utilizes guidelines appropriately.

Inappropriate staffing of a telephone nursing program can result in many problems. On one extreme, there are many licensed and nonlicensed nursing personnel making inappropriate clinical decisions. They may not have the necessary education, experience, or written guidelines (standing orders) that are all essential for safe patient care via the telephone. This creates an increased risk of errors of omission and commission, and thus an increased risk to the patient, nurse, and the organization.

On the other extreme, nursing personnel are too often used as messengers. This is an expensive, inefficient use of valuable personnel and time, and frequently results in multiple telephone calls and the dissatisfaction of all involved: caller, nurse, and physician.

For these reasons, it is recommended that telephone nurses who are responsible for clinical decisions be specially trained registered nurses. However, the approach and the information provided here can be of benefit to all personnel involved in ambulatory care.

A CALL FOR NEW LEVELS OF EXPERTISE

Telephone nursing is real nursing. It is not just triaging or referral, although these activities will often occur in interactions with "telephone patients." The telephone nurse and the patient, while physically distant, are still a nurse and a patient, and that relationship should maintain the same professional qualities on the telephone as it does in person. A nurse on the phone still bears the same responsibilities as a nurse in any other ambulatory setting, and the patient has the same needs. The differences between ambulatory-care nursing and telephone nursing lie in the limitations of the medium (the phone), which the nurse must work through to provide or ensure optimum care.

The availability of nursing expertise via the telephone gives patients (or "clients") a new level of service. They are able to:

- gain direct access to a professional nurse
- approach a complex health system in a simple manner, from their own homes, under the guidance of a sympathetic, knowledgeable listener
- discuss their health concerns and questions with a minimum of waiting time and at no cost
- find information and access to the appropriate level of care, from self-care procedures at home to emergency treatment, through nursing advice and referral
- address sensitive issues in relative anonymity, without the need for face-to-face interaction

The healthcare institution, as well as the patients, directly benefits from telephone nursing. High-quality telephone nursing:

- directs callers to the appropriate level of care for their specific problem, which assists organizations to provide cost-effective services
- assists in achieving continuity of care
- increases patient satisfaction

Today's healthcare consumers are seeking, and often demanding, more information about health and healthcare services. Many consumers, lacking a physician or not wishing to bother their physician after hours, perceive their only source of healthcare information and assistance to be the hospital emergency department. This results in many calls to the ER. The need for telephone nursing services places additional demands on already busy ER nurses, whose sophisticated skills are needed elsewhere in the department. The ER nurse, attempting to handle calls expediently and safely often recommends that all patients with concerns come to the ER. This leads to increased costs and the waste of valuable medical and nursing resources. Poor public relations can also result from this practice, as patients with non-urgent problems spend more and more time waiting for care in emergency departments.

Most ER nurses are trained and have expertise in "in person" nursing, with little emphasis on telephone nursing. They do not normally have access to the elements necessary to ensure good patient care via the phone: written telephone nursing guidelines, regular guideline reviews and updates, documentation procedures, quality assurance procedures, and "follow along" and follow-up procedures. In addition to improving the quality of telephone nursing provided, these guidelines and procedures protect the nurses and the organization from serious risks.

Telephone nursing, while using the same nursing skills needed to practice in-person nursing, requires new levels of expertise in a number of areas because of the limitations imposed upon the nurse by a phone interaction (see *Figure 3*). In short, the telephone nurse must excel in the use of the nursing process.

FIGURE 3. REQUIRED AREAS OF EXPERTISE FOR THE TELEPHONE NURSE

- **Active listening, with a clear and persuasive communication style**
- **Communication of both information and feelings without the benefit of eye contact, gestures, or props**
- **Establishment of a trusting relationship in a very short development of quick, accurate nursing assessments regarding the severity and urgency of caller concerns**
- **Creative problem solving, which requires identifying and mobilizing resources and providing appropriate information and referrals**
- **Identification and assurance of appropriate "follow along" and follow-up nursing activities**
- **Evaluation of care given to a patient via telephone nursing**

ROLES AND RESPONSIBILITIES

Patients call with a broad range of questions and concerns, the calls will reflect the diverse backgrounds of the callers. Many will simply need straightforward information, such as an appointment or a referral to a physician or clinic. These calls do not present much of a nursing challenge. However, many callers will need nursing care and expertise. Among the patient-care situations encountered in telephone nursing are:

- patients whose presenting complaint is not the "real" complaint
- patients whose presenting complaint is amenable to home care and/or physician-approved over-the-counter (OTC) drugs
- patients whose presenting complaint requires skilled nursing assessment and intervention
- patients who have been diagnosed by a physician and are seeking more information on this diagnosis, treatment options, or other matters
- patients who lack a regular physician and need a referral
- patients who need immediate or emergency care
- patients who require help gaining access to physicians or organizational programs
- patients with multiple concerns

The roles and responsibilities of the telephone nurse can be set forth in a clearly sequenced set of guidelines (see *Figure 4*). It should be kept in mind that the primary responsibility of the telephone nurse is *to assess the severity and the urgency of the problem* (not to provide a medical diagnosis nor to support the diagnosis assumed by the caller), and *to*

FIGURE 4. ROLES AND RESPONSIBILITIES OF THE TELEPHONE NURSE

- **Gather the information necessary to assess the problem.**
- **Working with the caller, define the caller's problem and the severity and urgency of that problem.**
- **Identify the appropriate resources, considering the characteristics of the caller, time of day, caller's access to resources, severity and urgency of problem, and other pertinent factors.**
- **Develop and suggest an appropriate plan of action: information referrals, follow-up, etc.**
- **Have the caller describe the actions he or she will take.**
- **Give the patient criteria with which to evaluate the outcomes of his or her actions.**
- **Establish evaluation criteria from a nursing-care perspective and evaluate outcomes.**
- **Document the call with as much information as possible, utilizing the "soap" format (subjective, objective, assessment, plan).**

give the appropriate advice for action, based on that assessment. The American Hospital Association classifies medical problems in the following manner (Mancini and Gale 1987):

- *Emergent* — Requires immediate medical attention. Delay is harmful to patient. The disorder is acute and potentially threatens life or function.
- *Urgent* — Requires medical attention within a few hours. The patient is in danger if not attended to. Disorder is acute but not necessarily severe.
- *Nonurgent* — Does not require the resources of an emergency service. The disorder is minor or nonacute.

All words, manners, and actions of the telephone nurse must take into consideration the limitations posed by the telephone (for example, lack of face-to-face contact and the information such contract provides). These limitations can be overcome by good communication skills, thorough assessment, creative problem solving, and accurate documentation (see *Figure 5*).

FIGURE 5. THE NURSING PROCESS: IN-PERSON v. VIA TELEPHONE

	IN-PERSON	VIA TELEPHONE
I. ASSESSMENT	Subjective and objective. Nurse uses all senses and can make objective assessment using all senses. Assess congruency of what patient says with what nurse experiences through other senses (general appearance, expressions, eye contact, mobility, odors, etc.) Can also use the insights of other professionals.	Mainly Subjective. Nurse is limited to auditory "clues" and actual words used. Objective only for tone of voice and speech patterns. Assess congruency of what patient says with what nurse hears. Limited to caller's interpretations.
II. PROBLEM DEFINITION OR NURSING DIAGNOSIS	Physical Environmental Psychological Health Behaviors	Physical Environmental Psychological Health Behaviors
III. PLANNING	Physical Care Education Consultation Referral	Physical Care Education Consultation Referral
IV. IMPLEMENTATION	Actual Care Education Consultation Collaboration	Education (Teach caller how to find care or provide self-care) Referrals Collaboration
V. EVALUATION	Nurse or other health provider evaluates.	Provide the means for the caller to evaluate.

SPECIAL PROBLEMS

Telephone nursing puts the nurse at a distinct disadvantage. He or she is asked to accurately assess the caller's problem and to provide triage and care, but is deprived of all visual cues. For this reason, the ability to listen on two levels (both to content and to emotion) becomes critical.

Because there are no visual cues for the nurse or the caller, several unique factors come into play:

- The nurse's ability to assess situation is challenged.
- The patient's ability to gauge response is limited, so the nurse must be careful about language and tone.
- There is no chart to examine.
- The nurse cannot use objective measurement (such as temperature) and is limited to information given by the caller, which by definition is subjective.

The nurse must use a "third ear," listening for clues other than the words spoken by the caller. Listening with a third ear involves active listening — integrating information and feelings into the knowledge base and conceptual framework of the professional nurse. The nurse must avoid letting the caller define the problem ("I have bronchitis") or its urgency ("I'm just having a little indigestion...it's not critical"). Gut reactions and intuitive abilities can be helpful in making accurate assessments and appropriate decisions under the circumstances.

Although somewhat handicapped by the telephone nursing situation, the nurse still is held accountable by the same professional, ethical, and legal standards that govern in-person nursing care. Because of these special problems, it is critical for the nurse to utilize the nursing process and be consistent with legal, professional, and organizational standards.

The nurse is not an unbiased listener. The unique background and ideas that each and every nurse brings to patient interactions must be recognized, as well as their influence on his or her approach to patient problems. The more different a nurse is from a patient, the more likely it is that communication problems and differing definitions will get in the way of successful interaction. Special ethical and legal issues must be kept in mind.

CONFIDENTIALITY. The contents of all telephone calls are to be held strictly confidential. Many callers may not be aware of the issue of confidentiality, so the nurse should inform them, especially in calls involving sensitive subjects such as substance abuse, reproductive issues, and sexually transmitted diseases.

PROFESSIONAL STATUS. The nurse must clearly communicate to the caller that his or her role is not to make a medical diagnosis but to provide appropriate information to the caller so that he or she can take appropriate action. It is the caller who makes the decisions.

SHARED RESPONSIBILITY. Both the caller and the nurse share in the responsibility for a productive interaction. The nurse is responsible for gathering information, being knowledgeable about health and a variety of illnesses, and communicating the scope of nursing practice. The nurse is also responsible for asking the caller what will be done about the problem, based on their information exchange. The caller is responsible for his or her feelings and actions, and communicating his needs and expectations.

LEGAL COMPLIANCE AND DOCUMENTATION. Nursing practice via the telephone must be in compliance with state laws governing nursing practice. In essence, professional nurses must not do medical diagnosis or medical procedures. In addition, there is a clear need for accurate documentation of the call; this serves to inform other caregivers and to represent correctly the advice or recommendations of the nurse. Thorough documentation is essential. From the standpoint of quality assurance and legal professionals, "If it isn't documented, it didn't happen."

USE OF PROTOCOLS OR GUIDELINES. Protocols, or telephone triaging and patient management guidelines, are provided to augment the education, expertise, and training of a registered nurse. They are not intended as fully complete guides to advice. Instead, they will alert the nurse to the general parameters of a caller's problem, suggest questions needed to make an accurate assessment, and provide care guidelines. Protocols or guidelines are only one resource, are not foolproof, and are not intended to supplant the expertise and experience of health professionals. Just as in any setting, these guidelines are only as good as the professional nurse who uses them. If the nurse goes down the wrong path and inappropriately assesses a situation, the guidelines cannot alert him or her of the problem. "Any person, institution, or organization using these guidelines assumes full responsibility for acts and omissions arising out of their use" (Group Health Cooperative of Puget Sound 1986, p.xii).

CHAPTER TWO

THE TELEPHONE NURSING PROCESS

Nurses are in the unique position of providing and facilitating appropriate, safe care via the telephone. Effective telephone nursing begins with the patient assessment process. The information necessary for a good assessment includes the data the caller provides as well as his or her perceptions of the problem or concern and degree of anxiety. Appropriate questioning by the nurse will further define the nature of the concern. During the phone interview, the nurse develops a sense of the urgency of the problem based upon objective and subjective information, including the nature of the complaint, the anxiety level of the caller, other existing medical conditions, and coexisting considerations (such as stress, anxiety, family problems, multiple medications, multiple problems, or language barriers). Following the nursing process, a systematic approach, the nurse uses this information to help the caller make decisions about the nature of the problem and develop a plan of action to address the problem (see *Figure 6*).

FIGURE 6.
THE NURSING PROCESS CYCLE

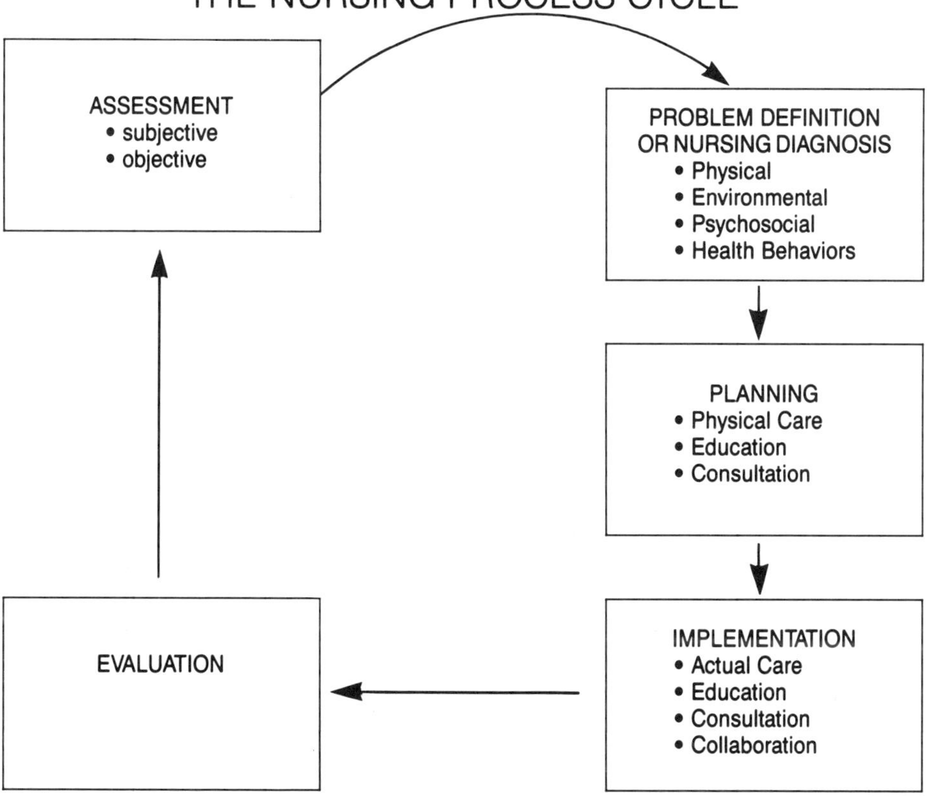

ASSESSMENT

The basis for all subsequent actions lies in gathering the type and amount of information necessary to make an accurate nursing assessment. This remains true whether the patient is presented in person or over the phone. To assess a patient a patient successfully, a nurse must possess specialized skills and knowledge, including:

- interviewing skills
- structured history-taking skills
- observation skills (in telephone nursing, "observation" equals "listening")
- physical assessment skills
- knowledge of pathophysiology
- knowledge of family, cultural, social, and psychological issues that might influence the patient's perception of the problem and intervention options

INTERVIEWING
Although the patient has instigated the visit or call, for many reasons he or she may not provide all the information necessary to make an accurate assessment.

- The patient does not share the same "language" (medical terminology) and usually lacks familiarity with specific body parts ("My stomach hurts" may refer to abdominal pain, epigastric pain, or chest pain). The definitions of the nurse may differ markedly from those of the caller.
- The patient may be embarrassed to discuss one or more aspects of the problem.
- The patient may have only a vague idea about what the problem is ("I just feel lousy").
- The patient may fear the personal consequences of a problem (such as in the case of substance abuse).

The nurse's first step is eliciting the chief complaint. As more information is revealed during the conversation, it may turn out that the original complaint is actually secondary to a larger or different problem, or was the caller's "excuse" for talking about a completely different concern. For example, a call about how to get rid of a hangover might turn into a call about drinking behavior. This is why attentive listening and the ability to wait for the caller's story to unfold are so important.

In essence, the nurse must determine the real reason for the call. The chief complaint should be documented as a short statement in the patient's own words, to include duration: "Sore throat, 3 days" or "Personal problems" for past month.

LISTENING

The interaction must be actively structured in such a way that trust is developed, and the caller is allowed to "tell his story."

START WITH OPEN-ENDED QUESTIONS. This lets the patient explain the problem in his or her own words. Closed questions (those requiring a yes or no answer) may affect the patient's choice of words and discourage elaboration. The nurse's comments should free the caller to provide more information, rather than prematurely narrowing the discussion to one symptom or topic. The following phrases are effective comments in the early stages of a conversation:

"Tell me more."
"Anything else?"
"Go on."

Once some information on the patient and the problem has been revealed, the nurse can choose to be more directive, as appropriate.

"Tell me how it started, and when."
"Did you have other similar problems?"

AVOID ASSUMPTIONS. When a nurse reacts negatively to a caller's statements, or as if he or she already knows what the problem is, the caller is put on the defensive and often discouraged from continuing. It should be kept in mind that many callers initially may be trying to determine if the nurse is a "safe" person with whom to discuss the real problem or concern.

CLARIFY. The patient who is confused or noncommittal sometimes must be encouraged to clarify his or her feelings through the use of gradually more directed questions. This is accomplished by tactfully clarifying the patient's answer to one question, and proceeding bit by bit from the general to the specific.

NURSE: "What is it that made you call tonight?"
PATIENT: "I just don't feel right."
NURSE: "You don't feel like your usual self?"
PATIENT: "That's for sure."
NURSE: "In what ways?"
PATIENT: "I'm awfully tired and dizzy lately."
NURSE: "First, tell me about your fatigue. When did it start?"

"How does it affect your life?"
"Now, tell me about your dizziness."

REFLECT THE PATIENT'S COMMENTS. Reflection helps the patient to provide more detail.

PATIENT: "The pain got worse and spread."
NURSE: "It spread . . ."
PATIENT: "Yes, to my arm. I thought I was going to die."
NURSE: "You were very frightened by the pain."

This technique helps to identify the specific content of the problem as well as the meaning of the problem to the patient.

HELP THE PATIENT TO FURTHER CLARIFY IDEAS. When a patient clarifies an idea, more information is being provided.

"Tell me what you mean by..."
"I didn't understand when you said..."

ASK ABOUT THE PATIENT'S FEELINGS. The nurse must not only inquire about the patient's feelings, but most acknowledge them and accept them.

"How did you feel when...happened?"
"It sounds like you were very upset."
"It sounds like it was depressing for you."

AVOID LANGUAGE THAT INFLUENCES DESCRIPTIONS. The patient's possible responses are limited when asked, "Is it a sharp or dull pain?" Instead the nurse should ask, "Can you describe the pain?"

ACCEPT DIFFERENT LEVELS OF "TALKATIVENESS." As with all people, some patients may be silent on the phone, and others may be overly talkative.

Silence can have several meanings. The silent caller:

- may be thinking carefully about a question. (Give him or her a minute to think through an answer. Don't think of silence as a vacuum that must be filled quickly with questions or comments.)
- may be angry, fearful, or suspicious of questions. (Speak calmly. Explain the importance of questions. Ask questions that get at the feelings behind the silence in a nonthreatening manner.)

- could be confused. (Restate the question using different words.)

A patient should not be labeled as uncooperative simply because he or she is silent. Silence can have many interpretations other than a negative one.

On the other hand, some callers may be so talkative that the nurse is not heard. Such a patient may be trying to avoid confronting anxiety by keeping the nurse at a distance. As long as the patient is the one talking, he or she may feel in control. This type of caller must be given some gentle feedback: "I feel concerned that you haven't heard me because you have so much to say. It's important to me that we understand each other. Let me restate what you've told me so far."

REMEMBER THAT THE CALLER'S VIEW OF THE NURSE IS CRITICAL. Telephone conversations go two ways. The caller is gathering information and making judgments just as the nurse is. If a nurse does not inspire trust, the caller will not be willing to share information. The caller may be asking himself or herself many questions during the course of a conversation.

- What information does this nurse want?
- Does this nurse care?
- Can I trust this nurse?
- Will the nurse tell my family or employer about my problem?
- Is the nurse really listening?
- What does he or she think of me and my problem?
- Will these people respond quickly if I need them?
- Am I talking with a real nurse and is he or she competent?

ASSESSING SYMPTOMS

In order to make a complete assessment of the patient's concerns, the nurse must obtain all of the following descriptive information:

- Patient age
- Symptom onset:
  1. Describe events occurring at the same time as the symptom began.
  2. Have there been similar episodes in the past?
  3. Did the symptom come on suddenly or gradually?
  4. How long did the symptom last?
- Location of symptom (anatomically precise)
- Character of symptom (for example, dull, sharp, or burning pain)
- Radiation of symptom

- Factors which precipitated or aggravated the symptom
- Factors which helped to stop or lessen the symptom
- Past evaluation, diagnosis, and treatment of the symptom:
  1. When, where, and by whom?
  2. What tests were performed in the past? What were the results of these tests?
  3. Was a diagnosis made? If so, what was the diagnosis?
  4. What treatment was given in the past? What was the result of this treatment? Present medications, allergies, pregnancy?
- Course of symptom (worse, better, same)
- Effect of symptom on normal daily activities

In order to elicit the most information from the patient, systematic guidelines should be followed when assessing symptoms, and all questions should be asked in an unbiased fashion (see *Figure 7*).

CONSIDERING THE HOLISTIC VIEW
Symptoms must be assessed within a holistic view of the patient. Florence Nightingale emphasized that the role of the nurse is to nurse the sick, not the sickness. A holistic focus includes consideration of the total individual. Some issues to explore are:

- family responsibilities
- living, work, and school conditions
- cultural beliefs
- financial issues
- lifestyle
- chronic and acute problems (health, social, and economic)
- health behaviors (health maintenance or crisis care, medications, medical regimens, habits such as smoking)

In sum, the patient is a complex individual influenced by family dynamics, the physical and social environment, cultural factors, and individual beliefs and attitudes.

PROBLEM DEFINITION

Once the necessary information on the patient has been gathered, a picture emerges. The synthesis of subjective and objective information results in nursing diagnoses or problem definitions that accurately describe the caller's problem or problems. Nursing diagnoses describe actual or potential health problems which nurses, by virtue of their education and experience, are capable and licensed to treat (Gordon 1982).

FIGURE 7. SYMPTOM ASSESSMENT

SYMPTOM CHARACTERISTICS	SAMPLE QUESTIONS TO ELICIT INFORMATION
1. ANATOMICAL LOCATION RADIATION OF SYMPTOMS	"Where does it hurt?" "Can you put your finger on it?" "Does the pain go anywhere?"
2. QUALITY OR CHARACTER	"What does it feel like?" "Can you compare this to something you have felt in the past?"
3. QUANTITY	"How severe or intense is the pain (on a scale of one to ten, ten being worst)?" "How much does it immobilize you?" "What effect does it have on your normal activities? Can you sleep?"
4. TIME SEQUENCE	"When did you first notice it?" "Is it constant?" "How long does it last?" "How often have you had it since that time?"
5. ENVIRONMENTAL FACTORS	"Where were you when it first occurred? What was going on?"
6. PRECIPITATING CONDITIONS	"Does it occur at a certain time of day?" "Is it related to eating, exercise, or any other activity?" "Does heat or cold seem to affect the pain?" "What appears to causes it?"
7. AGGRAVATING CONDITIONS	"Have you noticed anything that makes it worse?"
8. ALLEVIATING CONDITIONS	"What seems to help you feel better?"
9. CONCOMITANT SYMPTOMS	"Have you noticed any other changes present when you have the pain?"
10. REVIEW OF SYSTEMS	As appropriate.

Problem definition can be addressed by two complementary approaches: the problem-oriented approach and the nursing-diagnosis approach.

THE PROBLEM-ORIENTED APPROACH

The problem-oriented approach is accepted by medicine, nursing, and other health professions. It organizes the patient's problems for assessment, interventions, and ongoing care.

A problem is defined as any significant deviation that has influenced, is influencing, or may influence the patient's state of health or ability to function normally (Weed 1970). In a problem-oriented approach, the problems the nurse may encounter are not necessarily diagnoses. In fact, the initial entry on a problem list is quite often a sign, symptom, or a syndrome. The problem entered is the most specific that is possible at the time, defined in terms of exactly what is known about it — no more and no less. The list in *Figure 8* specifies various classes of patient problems, with examples.

FIGURE 8. CLASSES OF PATIENT PROBLEMS

(Sherman and Fields 1974)

CLASS OF PROBLEM	EXAMPLE
Proven diagnosis	Strep Pharyngitis
Physiologic entity	Congestive heart failure
Syndrome	Hyperventilation
Sign	Ankle edema
Symptom	Chest pain
Abnormal lab value	Elevated white blood cells
Allergy (environmental or drug)	Dust or penicillin
Drug sensitivity	Vomiting with antibiotic
Operation	Cholecystectomy
Risk factor	Smokes three packs of cigarettes per day
Psychological problem	Depression
Social problem	Unemployment

The format for documentation using the problem-oriented approach follows the "SOAP" outline:

- *Subjective* — the patient's observations, complaints, and past history (what the caller says)
- *Objective* — physical "finding," the tone and speech patterns heard by the nurse, background noises and breathing sounds
- *Assessment* — synthesis of the subjective and objective to define the problem (no medical diagnosis or terms unless previously diagnosed by a physician)
- *Plan* — referrals for services, resources, patient education, and follow-up

Subjective information is information that the caller gives to the nurse. Objective information can be seen, touched, smelled, tasted, or heard. Objective telephone nursing assessment utilizes the hearing sense only. To be considered objective, another person should also be able to experience the same sensation with their senses. Thus pain can never be objective.

If a number of problems are encountered during one call, each problem should be documented using the SOAP format (see Appendix E, "Nursing Assessment Worksheet and Tools"). The caller's problem may be a symptom combined with a health problem related to another factor, such as environment, life situation, or health behavior. This requires a creative problem-solving approach. It is important for the nurse to be able to slip out of problem-solving biases in order to help the caller come to the most appropriate and workable solution, given his or her own values, customs, and life situation (see *Figure 9*, "Become a Better Solution Generator").

Nurses possess a variety of resources that can be helpful in defining the caller's problem:

- symptom guides
- protocols
- their own knowledge and expertise
- the knowledge and expertise of their colleagues
- knowledge-based intuition — the synthesis of information

The first four resources are straightforward; the nurse can look in a book, think back to the last "similar" patient, consult with a colleague. The last resource, intuition, bears some explanation since it is an important and yet little-recognized resource for problem definition.

FIGURE 9. BECOME A BETTER SOLUTION GENERATOR

(Von Oech 1985)

Learn to recognize the ways that possible solutions are constrained.

VERTICAL THINKING

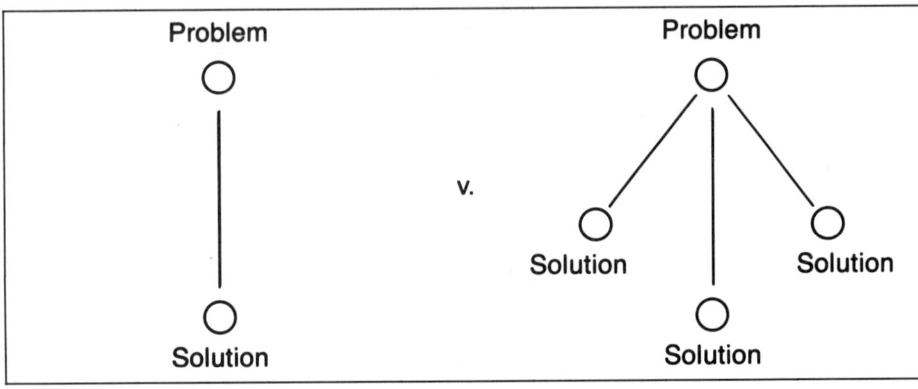

THINKING LANGUAGE

Symptom Diagnosis Prescription Treatment	v.	Problems Alternatives Interventions Solutions

STEREOTYPING

"That won't work— we've tried it before."	v.	"Every situation is different."

ARTIFICIAL CONSTRAINTS

Standard Operating Procedures: "We've always done it this way."	v.	"What would work best in this situation?"

LACK OF INQUISITIVENESS

"That's policy." "We always send them to the lab first."	v.	"Why does it have to be that way?" "Does the patient really need to do this?"

Intuition is a particularly valuable resource when problems are ambiguous, "fuzzy," complex, or unstructured. Intuition is generally thought of as a collection of guessing, feelings, and inspiration. It is denigrated by many, and is often associated with shoddy or lazy thinking. However, intuition, while it does not work in the same logical, linear progression as typical problem analysis, is of value because it is the synthesis of many kinds of information, all of which can contribute to an accurate nursing diagnosis.

Intuition can be thought of as "understanding without rationale" (Benners and Tanner 1987). Six aspects of intuitive judgment have been defined (Dreyfus 1985):

1. Pattern recognition and the ability to recognize relationships
2. Similarity recognition: the ability to recognize both similarities and dissimilarities
3. Common-sense understanding: a deep grasp of the real world and real people's responses to that world
4. Skilled know-how: true expertise — the ability to do something so well that it can be done in a wide variety of different situations
5. A sense of salience: the ability to extract the "truly important facts" from all the information at hand
6. Deliberative rationality: the ability to alter one's perspective and review all the facts from that new perspective

These aspects of intuitive judgment can work together to help the nurse synthesize information about a complex situation not amenable to "textbook solutions." They allow the nurse to define the problem accurately, so that all pertinent factors within the patient's life are taken into account.

THE NURSING-DIAGNOSIS APPROACH

Nursing diagnoses describe actual or potential health problems. These can be classified into four areas:

1. Physiological
2. Environmental
3. Psychological
4. Health behaviors (habits)

Nursing diagnoses differ from medical diagnoses. Although the two work together to define the entire range of problems the patient is experiencing, they define different aspects of the problem or problems (see *Figure 10*). These may be actual problems or perceived problems.

FIGURE 10.
DIFFERENCES BETWEEN MEDICAL DIAGNOSIS AND NURSING DIAGNOSIS

	MEDICAL DIAGNOSIS	NURSING DIAGNOSIS
Patient #1	Angina Pectoris	Chest Pain
Patient #2	Duodenal Ulcer	Altered Nutrition — less than body requirements, related to inability to ingest or digest food
Patient #3	Otitis Media	Ear Pain

A list of nursing diagnoses common to ambulatory-care settings is provided in *Figure 11*.

Nursing takes a holistic view of patients and their situations. Nurses are concerned about the broad range of responses people have to their environments and life situations. Nursing diagnoses can be organized by functional health patterns:

- health perception and health management
- nutrition and metabolism
- elimination
- activity (exercise)
- cognition (perception of situation)
- sleep and rest
- self-perception (self-concept)
- role relationships
- sexuality and reproduction
- coping (stress and tolerance)
- values and beliefs

Since these pattern areas are interdependent, a change in one area may be reflected in any or all other areas.

FIGURE 11.
NURSING DIAGNOSIS COMMON TO AMBULATORY CARE SETTINGS

Anxiety
Body Fluids, Alterations in
Bowel Elimination, Alterations in (constipation/diarrhea)
Breathing Patterns, Ineffective
Cardiac Output, Alteration in
Communication, Impaired Verbal
Consciousness, Altered Levels of
Coping Patterns, Maladaptive (individual)
Coping, Ineffective Family (compromised/disabling)
Digestion, Impairment of
Family Process, Inadequate
Fear (specify)
Fluid Volume Deficit
Grieving (anticipatory/dysfunctional)
Home Maintenance Management, Impaired
Injury, Potential for
Knowledge, Lack of (specify)
Manipulation
Mobility, Impairment of
Noncompliance (specify)
Nutritional Alteration (less/more than body requirements)
Pain
Parenting, Alterations in (actual/potential)
Respiratory Dysfunction
Role Disturbance
Self-Care Activities, Alterations in (specify feeding, bathing, hygiene)
Self-Concept, Alterations in (body image, self-image, self-esteem, role performance)
Sensory/Perceptual Alteration
Sexuality, Alteration in Patterns of
Skin Integrity, Impairment of (actual/potential)
Sleep/Rest Activity (disruption or arrhythmic)
Spirituality Matters (disruption of values or beliefs)
Social Isolation
Suffocation, Potential for
Thought Process, Impaired
Tissue Perfusion, Chronic Abnormal
Trauma, Potential for
Urinary Elimination, Impairment of
Verbal Communication, Impairment of
Violence, Potential for

PLANNING

The patient has been assessed. The problem has been defined. Now it is time for a plan of action (or a solution) to be created for the patient. This plan might include:

- an appointment
- a referral
- a self-care regimen or home-care plan
- a change in lifestyle or behavior
- a change in belief or knowledge
- an agreement to watch for further developments in symptoms and call back at a specified time

The best plans (or solutions) are created when all the factors within a patient's life are taken into account — not only the symptoms, but the resources on which the patient may draw, the factors which may make solving the problem difficult, and the beliefs or values he or she holds which may constrain possible solutions. Each patient is unique, and no "standard solution" is sufficient.

Developing a workable plan with a patient requires creativity: the ability to generate perhaps a number of alternatives to discuss with the patient. Alternatives encountering resistance may be modified or dropped altogether to ensure that the final plan is a realistic one that the patient can and will implement.

IMPLEMENTATION

Implementation includes the action taken by the nurse (such as referral, patient education, and follow-up) and the action taken by the patient. Follow-up calls by the nurse are an excellent means of assuring good patient care and the patient's compliance with recommended interventions. These calls also communicate that both the nurse and the organization truly care about the patient's health status and welfare.

EVALUATION

Evaluation includes a re-examination of each step in the nursing process:

- Was the appropriate assessment made?
- Was the problem definition correct?
- Was the plan appropriate?
- Was the implementation (or action) appropriate?

In essence, were the right things done? And were these "right things" done correctly? A complete evaluation brings the nursing process full cycle, back to the assessment stage, to re-assessment of the patient and the problem.

CHAPTER THREE

THE ART OF COMMUNICATING

Aside from clinical skills, the telephone nurse's most important skill is the ability to communicate: both to speak and to listen. Obviously, the ability to speak clearly, with the appropriate language and level of intimacy, is critical. The caller cannot benefit from the nurse's knowledge unless that knowledge is communicated. Equally important, however, is the nurse's ability to listen. The caller's problem cannot be accurately assessed and the right solutions recommended unless the nurse is able to hear the patient's "message," both spoken and unspoken. Every message "sent out" (via tone of voice, silence, gregariousness, or other means) communicates something. The nurse's goal is to communicate only what is intended, and that is accurate, empathetic nursing advice.

WORDS + EMOTIONS = MESSAGE

It is impossible to *not* communicate. No matter what is said or done, some message is communicated. If the tone of voice and the words used are not chosen with care, an unintended message may be communicated. Also, there are limits to the ways a nurse and a patient are able to communicate over the phone.

Sighted individuals rely heavily on visual clues to gather information, including signs that confirm or deny the meaning of the spoken word. The nurse who is limited to "seeing" patients over the phone must learn to gather information with the ears alone. Many auditory clues can be used to "check" the consistency between the words used and the way the caller sounds:

- pitch
- slowness or rapidity of speech
- unusual speech (slurred or confused, for example)
- laughter, groaning, moaning, or other exclamations
- breathing noises
- silence
- background noises

Does the sound of the patient's voice match what he or she is saying?

Emotional clues may also be valuable. The nurse's own feelings, in response to the caller's words or tone of voice, can serve to clarify the patient's situation. If a nurse feels sad, angry, or afraid, a clear (although unspoken) message has been communicated.

In addition to being limited to receiving messages by hearing only, the telephone nurse is limited to expressing messages by speaking only. In-person interactions can involve eye contact, gestures, and sometimes physical contact, but phone interactions, by their very nature, cannot. The nurse must develop a telephone personality which projects the qualities consumers expect to find in a healthcare professional: competence, caring, and accessibility.

Simple telephone courtesy must also be a part of the nurse's manner.

- There should be no excessive waiting.
- Prompt follow-up and call-backs are essential when consultation with colleagues is required.
- Clear expectations should be set and followed: "I must check on that. I will call you back in ten minutes."

ESTABLISHING TRUSTWORTHINESS

To facilitate positive communication, the nurse must work to create a feeling of trustworthiness. The nurse's voice, manner, and words must help to build a relationship the caller. Trust is based on consistency, respect, and sensitivity.

CONSISTENCY. Nursing style should be consistent with interpersonal style and consistent over time. Many brusque people still manage to convey warmth, and "mushiness" is not a prerequisite to caring. The words used should come from within, not from a book or a fellow nurse. In the same way, a nurse's style should not vary dramatically from call to call. This is especially critical during call-backs and follow-ups.

RESPECT. The nurse who wishes to gain the trust of a caller must show respect for that person: his or her opinions, concerns, and feelings. Demonstrated interest in what the caller has to say is essential.

SENSITIVITY. Sharing sensitivity involves being aware of and responding to the cues given by the speaker — and those given by the nurse as well. In telephone nursing, these cues include tone of voice, slowness or rapidity of speech, silence, and hesitation. It is also important to speak to the caller at the appropriate level of intimacy. When callers discuss health issues with a nurse, they do not want to talk to a "friend," but to a friendly professional nurse.

ACTIVE LISTENING

It takes two to speak the truth:
one to speak, and another to hear.
Henry David Thoreau

Active listening refers to behaviors which help to elicit, support, and clarify the speaker's message. Active listening can be useful to telephone nurses to demonstrate interest in a speaker and thus build trust and openness. It is also useful in clarifying the speaker's message and facilitating accurate communication, sharing not only ideas but the feelings behind the ideas.

There are two levels to all that we say: the literal meaning of our words and the emotional content (or the "message behind the message"). While listening to a caller, the nurse must focus not only on factual content but on what is implied or even left unsaid by the speaker.

"Mirroring," an active listening technique, can help to clarify the content of messages. It simply involves repetition of the caller's message by the nurse. Mirroring clarifies the caller's true meaning, demonstrates listening, and confirms that the listener understands. It also allows the speaker to hear the words he or she used and rephrase, if necessary, to get the correct message across.

PATIENT: "My knee hurts."
NURSE: "Your knee hurts?"
PATIENT: "Well, it's not my knee actually....I guess it's just my whole leg. I can't put any weight on it."

Rephrasing is another useful active listening technique. Here, the nurse puts the speaker's message into other words, thus testing understanding. When a message is rephrased, nuances of meaning are added. This technique is very valuable in situations where a nurse is dependent upon the information provided by the patient (such as during assessment).

It is beneficial to use different words than the speaker to ensure a precise understanding of the message. *Figure 12* provides a list of useful synonyms for telephone nursing.

Reflective listening skills can be used to demonstrate listening and understanding, whether the speaker is a patient, friend, or supervisor. These skills are also helpful in clarifying information, especially when a patient provides information that is vague or difficult to follow.

FIGURE 12.
USEFUL SYNONYMS FOR TELEPHONE NURSING

FEAR	**Frightened, terrorized, anxious, have misgivings, concerned, feel a sense of dread, alarmed, apprehensive, worried.**
ANGER	**Frustrated, offended, resentful, bitter, hostile, displeased, injured, insulted.**
SADNESS	**Depressed, overwhelmed, rejected, defeated, unhappy, mournful, anguished.**
CONFUSION	**Mixed up, don't understand, can't remember, forgot.**
HAPPINESS	**Relieved, comfortable, okay, glad, satisfied, content, feel lucky, pleased.**

Examples of reflective statements include:

"As I understand you..."
"In other words..."
"So, you mean that..."
"I'm hearing that..."

In each case, the listener is attempting to reflect accurately back to the speaker the message that has been received. It is usually more useful to reflect the message in a way that demonstrates understanding of the message.

PATIENT: "My head really hurts."
NURSE: "You have a headache."

In this instance, the nurse has shown the patient that the message has been received. The message has not, however, been clarified (What kind of pain? Where is the worst pain?). This is in contrast to the following approach:

PATIENT: "My head really hurts."
NURSE: "So you're having a lot of pain, in your head?"
PATIENT: "I don't think it's a migraine....I drank a little too much last night."

NURSE: "As I understand it then, you need some help in treating your headache, which you think might be a hangover?"
PATIENT: "Yes, but not only that....I'm a little concerned about the way that drinking makes me feel. I mean, how much is too much?"
NURSE: "It sounds like you'd like to talk about how drinking is affecting you."

This approach, if handled well, can produce the same results as the first — the speaker still feels as though he or she has been heard. It has the added benefit of eliciting a great deal of information.

The nurse should be aware of some potential problems with this approach. The reflective listener must maintain a flexible stance when rephrasing a remark because there is always a possibility that the speaker's message is being misinterpreted. The speaker must feel comfortable saying, "No, that's not what I meant." Also, some people use this technique as a way of telling the other person how they feel, rather than simply rephrasing the message. This can leave the caller feeling defensive. Psychoanalysis is best left to psychoanalysts, and the nurse should concentrate on the content of the message.

Figure 13 provides a summary of active listening skills, factors, and techniques.

DEALING WITH EMOTIONS

There are two people involved in every telephone nursing interaction: the nurse and the patient. While it is sometimes easier to focus attention on the communication style and responses of the patient when emotion comes into the picture, it is unwise to ignore the nurse's personal role in the interaction.

Perhaps one of the most useful stances for the nurse to maintain when dealing with an emotional caller is to use descriptive, rather than valuative statements. The nurse's emotional reaction should be minimized as much as possible, since anger, anxiety, or sadness will most likely not help the caller (although this emotional state can provide information about the caller's problem, especially if the caller is denying the problem). Allowing the caller to vent emotion may sometimes calm him or her down enough to carry on a productive interaction.

The nurse's ability to handle the caller's feelings, negative or otherwise, may engender feelings of personal trust and professional confidence. A

FIGURE 13. ACTIVE LISTENING SKILLS
(Botton 1979)

SKILL	FACTORS AND TECHNIQUES
ATTENDING	Minimizing distractions Attentiveness Body language (which influences tone of voice) Concentration
"FOLLOWING"	Attentive silence Words to help start and prolong conversation Infrequent (noninterrupting) questions
REFLECTION	Clarifying Paraphrasing "Feeling" words Summarizing
"NONWORD" COMMUNICATION	Tone of voice Rapidity of speech
ATTITUDE	Empathy Acceptance Assertiveness ("I")

problem-solving orientation provides the caller with an opportunity to save face in situations where he or she might actually be a part of the problem. "Drugs are very damaging to your health" is a problem-oriented statement; "You are a drug addict" is a person-oriented statement. A person with a potential drug abuse problem is more likely to be receptive to the first approach.

The nurse must be ever mindful of the fact that the caller takes a risk by calling, even if that risk may appear low. It is important to respond to the caller in such a way that he or she feels valued. A nurse can demonstrate respect by responding with phrases and a tone of voice which:

- recognize the caller's existence
- recognize the caller's uniqueness as an individual, rather than his or her role as a part of the job

- acknowledge the caller's worth as a person
- acknowledge that the caller's problem is viewed seriously
- acknowledge the validity of the caller's perception of the world
- demonstrate a willingness to be involved with the caller, at least for the duration of the call

THE DIFFICULT CALLER

Although nurses do their best to be supportive listeners and speakers, there will be callers who evoke frustration, depression, or anger. Some of these difficult callers may be easy to handle; others may be intimidating because the nurse is not sure exactly how to approach them.

ANGRY CALLER. A caller may be angry for a variety of reasons. The telephone nurse, for example, may be the sixth person the caller has talked to about a problem, and patience may have run out with the fifth person. Or, the caller may be angry about experiencing the problem, and the telephone nurse may be the only one around on whom this anger can be vent. The caller may have unrealistic expectations about the nurse's ability to solve the problem. If these expectations continue, even if they are unrealistic, there will be continued anger. There are, however, steps the telephone nurse can take to defuse anger in a caller.

1. Introduce yourself, your position, and your willingness to help. You are in the position of "expert authority." Your willingness to listen and help validates the importance of the caller and his or her requests. "I'm Mary Jones, the head nurse. How can I help?"

2. Listen. This tells the caller that he or she has your undivided attention. Let the person tell you his or her story. This may include expectations that have not been met by the system or by a particular person. Note the content of the caller's concerns. Avoid interrupting.

3. Acknowledge anger or anxiety one time only — initially. Tell the person that the feeling (anger, anxiety, or whatever) has been adequately conveyed to you. Use phrases such as : "It sounds like you're really upset about..."

4. Focus on the content of the caller's expectations. Continue to focus on facts, not angry feelings. Avoid raising your voice. Be descriptive; ask clarifying questions. "Mirror" the person's own statements of content: put his or her words in your mouth. This

lets the person know you are listening, understanding, and caring; it allows the person to "see" and hear himself or herself.

5. Summarize the content of the caller's expectations. Continue to gather and provide information concerning content items (such as person, place, time, system). "So let me see if I have all the information. You think that you need a refill on your prescription and that you need this today."

6. Prioritize the person's expectations. Make sure that you both agree on the priorities so that expectations can be met. "So you are saying that you think it is most important that..."

7. Offer choices that will meet the priorities. These choices often will involve creative problem-solving. The caller may not be able to get everything (person, place, time, and system) in the exact configuration desired. For example, if time is the priority, you might say, "I can do my best to see that someone, somewhere does that today." Or, if the person and not time is the priority, you might say, "I can do my best to see that Dr. Holloway calls you as soon as she's available." Check the acceptability of the alternatives to the caller: "How does that sound to you?"

8. Continue to "follow" the person until his or her needs are met or until another health professional assumes responsibility. This action avoids "person abandonment" into the system. If the situation changes, the patient still has contact with the system. "Please call me on Monday and let me know if things are working out for you. Ask for me personally."

PLEASING CALLER. This caller wants to give all the "right" answers. His or her goals is to please the nurse, so the answers provided are whatever the caller thinks the nurse wants to hear.

ANXIOUS CALLER. Fear or anxiety can get in the way of an accurate assessment. Even when a problem is minor, it may not be possible to reassure an anxious caller.

KNOW-IT-ALL CALLER. Why does the "know-it-all" bother to call when he or she is already such a medical expert? It can be very difficult to assess such a patient, as he or she has already "self-diagnosed."

DEPRESSED CALLER. When a caller is feeling depressed, this emotional state may interfere with the ability to assess his or her health status accurately or to report the range of feelings or their cause. It is important to ascertain that this patient is not suicidal.

MANIPULATIVE CALLER. During a conversation with a manipulative caller, the nurse may begin to feel "used." Whether the request is for an inappropriate prescription or a validation of maladaptive behavior, this caller is out to get something that is not really offered by the telephone nurse.

UNREALISTIC CALLER. The unrealistic caller usually wants the nurse to "fix it." He or she is not satisfied when the limits of a nurse's legal or ethical abilities to address the problem have been reached.

PASSIVE OR UNRESPONSIVE CALLER. The passive caller does not hold up his or her end of the telephone conversation. Although there are two persons interacting, it may seem like just one is trying to solve the problem (the nurse).

SUICIDAL CALLER. This caller states that he or she is seriously contemplating suicide. The nurse may have no evidence to prove that this will not occur. The one "hope" is that he or she cared enough to call.

OBSCENE CALLER. The obscene caller is clearly abusive and manipulative. While "obscenity" normally refers to sexual obscenity, any abusive caller is obscene.

DENYING CALLER. Although this caller has called to discuss some problem, he or she is not willing to discuss the real problem (such as an unhealthy habit or behavior). Or the caller may be too frightened to consider that the problem is serious (for example, chest pains indicative of a cardiac problem may be dismissed as "gas").

Telephone nursing can be stressful. The number and kind of calls are unpredictable, and the nurse may encounter personal "negative" emotions while engaged in telephone nursing. Being aware of the risks to one's own emotional health can help the nurse to create adaptive patterns with which to address these risks.

PATIENT PERSUASION AND EDUCATION

It is simply not enough to provide accurate information and to develop an effective nursing plan to solve or ease the caller's problem. The telephone nurse must also persuade the patient to accept assessment and advice. This may include: (1) convincing the caller of the nurse's sincerity, competence, and expertise; (2) providing education about health issues, medications, symptoms, and other related matters; and (3) motivating the patient to change.

Before a nurse can become a credible source of information for the patient, the patient's trust must be won — in the nurse as a professional and as a person who is on his or her side. As in all settings, a primary role of the nurse is *patient advocate*. Should the caller come to feel that a nurse has a personal "agenda" to pursue, rather than his or her best interests at heart, the caller's goodwill will have been lost and the nurse will be unable to influence him or her. In the same way, the caller must be convinced of the nurse's professional abilities. An intelligent and caring manner, the questions asked, and sensitivity to individuality and concerns will convince a caller that a nurse knows what he or she is doing. Once the nurse/patient relationship is started, the teaching can begin.

Patients have a need for education on many levels:

- specific instructions (such as restating the physician's advice; telling a patient what the pre-lab test protocol is, or giving directions regarding organizational services)
- explanation of illness processes (such as telling the caller what to look for and when to be concerned, or reassuring the caller when the symptoms are not usually indicative of the illness he or she fears)
- teaching new health behaviors (such as better exercise habits; how to implement dietary changes successfully)
- challenging incorrect beliefs or maladaptive behaviors (such as explaining the risks posed by substance abuse or correcting patient's misinformation about illnesses, medications, or treatments)

When an attempt is made to change the behavior of any person, there is an implied criticism: the person is doing the "wrong" thing, and thus should change. Few people are able to change easily. The more deeply the person holds a feeling behind a behavior, the more difficult it is to change that behavior.

When trying to make a caller aware of the need to change, it is important to keep the patient's point of view in mind. The nurse should think about why the patient is engaging in the behavior. What does it do for him or her? Is it related to a value, attitude, or belief held by the patient? If the behavior is based on a value, it will be difficult to change. If the behavior is based on a mistaken belief, however, it may be possible to help the patient to change by simply providing new or correct information. Beliefs are based on fact (correct or incorrect). Attitudes are more transitory than values, and they can be changed with new information. Because they grow out of values, attitudes are more consistent than beliefs. Values are deeply held and are stable over time; they are quite difficult to change.

FIGURE 14. UNDERSTANDING BELIEFS, ATTITUDES, AND VALUES BEHIND PATIENT BEHAVIORS

	PATIENT #1	PATIENT #2
OBSERVABLE BEHAVIOR	Is not regularly using birth control; is at risk for unwanted pregnancy	Is not regularly using birth control; is at risk for unwanted pregnancy.
BELIEFS	"It's okay to use 'coitus interruptus.' Anyway, no birth control method is foolproof."	"You can't get pregnant if you 'do it' only once in a while."
ATTITUDE	"I don't really think about it."	"You shouldn't plan on having sex. If you are 'swept away' and it 'just happens,' it's much better than if you premeditatively decided to do it."
VALUE	Premarital sex is okay.	Premarital sex is wrong.

Figure 14 provides examples of the relationship between observable behaviors and beliefs, attitudes, and values. While both patients in the examples are engaging in similar behaviors, they are doing so for different reasons. Each will need to receive (and believe) a different set of information in order to begin to change that behavior.

Nurses must choose their battles carefully and attempt to change only those behaviors that are changeable about their patients. For example, if a patient is at high risk for arteriosclerotic heart disease and is a heavy smoker with unhealthy eating habits, he or she will most likely try to change only one of these behaviors. The largest benefit to this particular patient will probably come from stopping smoking. To suggest changing all unhealthy behaviors is to risk alienating the patient and losing those positive behavioral changes that could have occurred had the relationship been preserved. One sensitive approach is to offer the patient information on the benefits associated with the "cost" of change for each behavior.

It is not enough that the nurse or the physician believes the patient should change. The patient needs to believe that the behavioral change will offer sufficient reward for the effort of changing.

Nurses commonly would like to change the following patient behaviors:

- smoking
- overeating or undereating
- unhealthy nutritional habits
- substance abuse
- noncompliance with prescribed medical regimens (for example, patient will not take prescribed medications as instructed or will not follow recommended actions, such as diagnostic tests or treatments)

Thinking about why the patient engages in a behavior is useful in assessing how to approach persuading and educating the patient. What does the behavior do for the patient? Will the new behavior do the same thing? Is there a period of sacrifice necessary before the "good" behavior feels as good as the "bad" behavior? For example, patients sometimes do not take prescribed medications as instructed. This may be because they do not like to take medication or feel they do not need as much as was prescribed; they may find it too expensive and not even buy it; or they may be confused about the reason for the medication. The nurse must seek to understand the reason for the behavior before persuasion of the patient is approached.

There is no question about it — it is difficult to change a patient's behavior. The implied criticism that accompanies the call for change is difficult for the patient to accept as well. It is therefore important for the nurse to impart the message that change is necessary with as much sensitivity for the person's feelings as possible.

The "sensitive line" is the point at which individuals become defensive and protective of themselves in the face of information that disagrees with their own self-image. A continuum of patient descriptors, based on the opinions of four nurses, is provided in *Figure 15*. Clearly, nurses #3 and #4, were they to voice their feelings, would pass the sensitive line beyond which the caller would feel unfairly criticized. Their statements could destroy the tentative relationship between the caller and the nurse. Sometimes, however, it is necessary to convey information which is difficult to hear.

FIGURE 15.
CONTINUUM OF PATIENT DESCRIPTORS

Patient's Self-Image: "I believe it is important to attempt to get what you want out of life. When I called the nurse, I clearly requested what I wanted."

Nurses' Reactions:

NURSE #1: "This patient was easy to deal with because she knew what she wanted."
NURSE #2: "This patient was very assertive."
NURSE #3: "This patient was pushy."
NURSE #4: "This patient was very difficult. She was selfish and only focused on her own needs."

#1	#2	#3	#4
Straightforward	Assertive	Pushy	Very Difficult

What happens if there is a need to communicate information which is beyond the sensitive line? Nurses must take care to provide feedback which is:

- *verifiable* (can be objectively checked)
  "Your voice is raised."
  "Alcohol destroys brain cells."

- *predictable* (received at a logical point in the interaction)
  "When you raise your voice like that, I have to interrupt you. I need you to not yell at me when you tell me that you want...."
  "Once again, when you mention 'partying,' I get the feeling that you feel a little out of control."

- *controllable* (caller decides level of criticism to receive)
  "Once again, I need to speak with you about your yelling. Can we please focus on that for a moment?"
  "I think it would be a good idea to talk about your use of alcohol. Would you like to discuss that?"

The nurse's intelligent and caring manner, and sensitivity to concerns, especially when there is a need to convey potentially offensive information, will help to create a setting in which an effective nurse/patient relationship can develop.

CHAPTER FOUR

SPECIAL PATIENT POPULATIONS

Although the term "development" is typically associated with the young, human beings continue to grow through different developmental phases throughout their lifespan. Each stage of life involves dealing with different issues. It is important to keep these stages in mind when speaking with patients, as these life issues subject the individual to different health risks and stresses, and lend him or her different strengths with which to achieve and maintain health. Cultural issues, too, present special health concerns, and nurses must be sensitive to diverse beliefs and values if optimal care is to be provided.

INFANTS AND CHILDREN

In pediatrics more than any other specialty, telephone contact has become an important component of patient care. The lack of extended family support, combined with the likelihood of mothers working outside the home, has expanded the roles of physicians and pediatric health professionals in the family. Mothers today may call their children's physician's office with questions that, a generation ago, they might have asked their mothers or aunts.

Although mothers wish more contact with the physician, they often lack time to spend in waiting rooms and are thus interested in telephone access to advice. It has been estimated that 60 percent of all patient contacts with pediatric offices are via the telephone. Because many mothers are uncomfortable calling the physician on "minor" topics that are nonetheless of concern to them, Nurse on Call nurses are sure to receive calls about children's illnesses and parents' concerns about infant and child behavior.

Telephone pediatric contact is complicated by the fact that the nurse is always speaking to a third party (the parent or other caregiver) and therefore does not have the benefit of listening to the patient's voice and hearing the patient's actual description of the condition. This can make telephone assessment and triage more difficult for the nurse. Most times it is best to "take the caller's temperature" with regard to perception of the severity and urgency of the problem (J. Brown 1989). This can be accomplished by following these steps:

- Assess the level of anxiety being experienced by the parent: "Do you feel frightened by the way your child looks or is behaving?" Sometimes parents call just for reassurance that their child is not seriously ill or that his or her behavior is not developmentally unusual.
- Assess how the child actually looks and is behaving: "Does

your child look much sicker than he has in the past with a cold? In what way? What has he been doing for the past four hours?"
- Determine the reason for the call at this particular time (rather than earlier or later). "Did something about your child's condition change?"

In any event, the nurse should trust personal feelings and the perceptions of the parents. "Both your intuition and the parent's should never be disregarded when you are deciding whether a patient should be seen immediately" (J. Brown 1989, p.7).

If the assessment is that the patient does not need to be seen in the emergency room or by a physician at the present time, the parents must be informed about what to expect from the illness:

- how long symptoms (such as fever or vomiting) may last
- when to call back for more information or guidance ("If Johnny is still vomiting in two hours, call me back or contact your physician.")
- whether the illness is contagious
- warning signs that would change the nonurgent assessment

The caller should always be told when and how they can obtain immediate care, should they feel the need to do so.

There are specific risks associated with the population of infants and children:

SUDDEN INFANT DEATH SYNDROME (SIDS). SIDS is a leading cause of infant death in the United States, claiming approximately 15,000 infants per year (Edelman and Mendel 1986). Its onset is unexpected and, at present, unexplainable. This creates a great deal of anxiety for parents. Highest incidence is between one and eight months of age.

AUTOMOBILE ACCIDENTS. An infant not securely strapped into an approved carseat is at risk for serious injury or death from even the most minor car accidents (or "fender benders"). No infant or child should be inside a car without being strapped into an approved carseat. Children should remain in a carseat until they weigh forty pounds or more. At forty pounds, a seatbelt can provide protection. Both shoulder and lap belts should be used, even in the back seat.

ASPIRATION OF FOREIGN OBJECTS AND DANGEROUS SUBSTANCES. Infants learn about the world by physical and visual exploration. One of the baby's primary "exploratory devices" is his or her mouth. Everything goes in a baby's mouth, which is why infants are at such a high risk for ingesting poisons and aspirating harmful foreign objects. Parents should be counseled to keep all small or dangerous objects away from the baby. "Babyproofing" should be completed throughout the infant's physical environment by the time that baby is ready to make the leap into movement. Poisons can include agents not considered dangerous to adults, or substances that adults would not notice as posing a threat to themselves: plants, food additives, medicines (OTC and prescription drugs), chemicals, alcohol, cleaning agents, old paint chips from trim and walls (may contain lead), and more.

ABUSE. "In most abusive families, abuse begins in infancy" (Gallagher and Kreidler 1987). Abuse may be verbal, physical, emotional, sexual, or a combination of the four. Abuse is devastating to the infant's need to establish trust and build the foundation for future relationships with others. The violation of this trust through abuse can put the infant or child at risk for a variety of health and emotional problems which may last for the rest of his or her life. It is therefore imperative that high-risk families be identified prior to or early in the cycle of abuse. Suspicions of child abuse should be reported immediately, and parents should be referred to organizations that can help them deal with their feelings in ways not detrimental to their children (such as Parents Anonymous). In many states, it is required by law that nurses report all suspected cases of child abuse.

FALLS. Both infants and children are at risk for falls which can cause serious injury or even death. Young infants often fall from heights, such as tabletops, because the parents do not realize the movement capacities of even the tiniest baby. Toddlers and older children are curious and daring, and put themselves in dangerous situations. They are prone to misjudge their own abilities and the potential dangers of a situation. Parents should be advised to install safety railings at the tops and bottoms of all stairways in their home. Crib railings should be kept up to keep the baby inside the crib, and even tiny infants are best left on the floor, where their movements will not result in falls.

BURNS. Risks of burns to the infant can be minimized by keeping the baby away from heat-producing items such as fireplaces, humidifiers, radiators, candles, matches, cigarettes, and lighters. All electrical outlets should be covered, and babies should be taught early that outlets and electrical cords are "no-no's." If possible, infants and young children should be kept out of the kitchen; this will remove them not only from proximity to the stove, but from a variety of other dangerous items such as knives, cleaning fluids, and electrical appliances. Older children should be taught fire safety rules, and adults using the stove should turn all pot handles toward the back of the stove to avoid scalding spills.

FLU, VIRUSES, AND OTHER BIOLOGICAL AGENTS. Infants who attend daycare are at high risk for infectious illness. Contagious diseases pass from infant to infant via playthings, as well as from caregivers to infants. Although most daycare facilities have rules against children attending while ill, many infections are passed prior to the appearance of symptoms. Because children under two have immature eustachian tubes, they are prone to middle ear infections (otitis media). Both infants and children should be immunized against serious childhood illnesses according to recommended immunization schedules.

DROWNING. Although it is common sense that infants and children should never be left unsupervised around water, drowning is a leading cause of death in this age group. Infants are completely helpless in water and can easily drown in even a tiny amount of water. They should never be left alone in a baby bath, bathtub, or wading pool for any reason. Dozens of infants and toddlers drown each year in toilets, mop buckets, and other unexpected places. Children should be taught water safety, including how to float, as soon as they are old enough to understand such instruction. Toilets should be left closed at all times, as they present a drowning risk to toddlers.

ADOLESCENTS

The adolescent is at a vulnerable and critical developmental stage. While not yet possessing the maturity to make adult decisions, the adolescent possesses the ability to engage in behaviors which may affect his or her adult life. Adolescence is, for many people, the first time in their lives they are exposed to "adult" concerns: alcohol and drug use; sexuality; intense and adult-like relationships; access to automobiles, motorcycles, and mass-transit without adult supervision; and new family and social roles. The adolescent's social world expands increasingly away from the family, and peers take on critical importance. This is a time of crisis ("danger and opportunity") for both the adolescent and the family, as each struggles to adjust to the inevitable changes that growth and maturation brings.

Areas of health-related concern are:

SEXUALITY. Although a large percentage (30 to 50 percent) of teenagers become sexually active before their eighteenth birthday, adolescent sexuality is not often dealt with realistically by teenagers or their parents. Many teenagers are unwilling or unable to take responsibility for their own behavior (specifically in the area of birth control), and many parents are loathe to discuss proactively with their teenagers the realities of sexual behavior. The teenager's lack of knowledge and experience, combined with irresponsibility and a lack of communication (especially between teenage partners) puts him or her at risk for sexually transmitted diseases, unwanted pregnancy, and psychosocial problems (such as promiscuity, confusion, or guilt).

PREGNANCY. There is an alarmingly high rate of teenage pregnancy in the United States. Each year, more than one million teenage girls become pregnant; one-half are not married. In addition to the obvious economic and social risks posed by such pregnancies, there are significant physical ones as well. Those under age fourteen are at high risk for toxemia, prolonged labor, and postpartum complications. Their infants are at risk for prematurity and low birth weight. Critical to the teenage mother and her infant are early diagnosis, good nutrition, and close monitoring throughout pregnancy.

ALCOHOL AND DRUG USE. Because of alcohol's role in accidental death, especially auto accidents, alcohol use may represent the single biggest threat to an adolescent's life. Drug use, while less prevalent than alcohol use, is still a major threat to this population. Tobacco, also an addictive and physically damaging drug, is widely used by this group, and young females represent the single "growth" population for cigarette use. There are many health problems, injuries, and fatalities associated with alcohol abuse:

- *automobile accidents* — 50 percent of all automobile accidents involve alcohol (Banker, Burton, and Zieve 1986)
- *suicide* — over 60 percent of fatal accidents and suicides involve alcohol use
- *fire deaths* — 50 percent of fatalities involve alcohol
- *choking on foods* — 25 percent of incidences involve alcohol
- *freezing to death* — 20 percent of fatalities involve alcohol
- *drowning* — 20 percent of fatalities involve alcohol
- *accidental asphyxiation* — 20 percent of fatalities involve alcohol
- *falls* — 20 percent of fatalities involve alcohol
- *violent crimes* — 70 percent of all violent crimes involve alcohol (Murray and Zentner 1985)

AUTOMOBILE ACCIDENTS. Automobile accidents are the leading cause of death among adolescents. As previously mentioned, alcohol use figures prominently in this grim statistic.

SUICIDE. Over 14 percent of those aged fifteen to twenty-four who died in 1986 did so by their own hand. Suicide is the third leading cause of death in this age group. It is important to openly discuss suicide with anyone who "hints" at it. A simple question, "Are you thinking of killing yourself?" can open the door for a desperate person to discuss their feelings. Those who are considering suicide will often be willing to talk about it, and appropriate resources can be mobilized.

YOUNG ADULTS

The "young adult" is defined here as a person between the ages of eighteen and twenty-five who is experiencing the developmental stresses and life situations appropriate to that age group. Young adults have special needs and engage in unique behaviors, and these must be recognized by the nurse in order to assess problems accurately and recommend appropriate healthcare solutions. This stage of development makes the individual vulnerable to certain stresses which can have a substantial impact on health status. Young adults often engage in high-risk behaviors, such as experimentation with drugs, and these can have far-reaching effects on their future lives.

Important developmental tasks for this age group include (Murray and Zentner 1985):

- establishment of a stable identity, including sexual identity
- attainment of independence from family
- selection of future occupation and development of work-related skills and abilities
- acceptance of body form and function
- establishment of first sexual relationships
- clarification of value system, philosophy, and standards of behavior

Special health risks to this population occur in these areas:

HEALTH PERCEPTION AND HEALTH MANAGEMENT. Most young adults consider themselves healthy and are inexperienced with health problems and the healthcare system. Many view themselves as invincible and invulnerable to health problems. They will view any and all symptoms within the context of their culture, developmental stage, and the experience of others. They also view symptoms within their current demands in life. In the past, management of health issues of young adults has usually been addressed by someone other than a health professional (parents, for example).

NUTRITIONAL AND METABOLIC CONCERNS. Many young adults do not eat properly. This includes inappropriate quality and quantity of food. They also eat at erratic times and often eat "junk food." This population (especially the women) is at risk for eating disorders such as anorexia and bulimia.

ACTIVITY LEVELS AND EXERCISE. Young adults often encounter problems managing the quality and quantity of physical exercise. These problems range from the person who engages in no regular exercise and may experience lethargy, to those who are "weekend warriors" and engage in strenuous activities periodically, resulting in problems related to overuse or inappropriate use of unconditioned bodies.

SLEEP. Young adults are particularly notorious for erratic sleeping habits: "all nighters" for study or "all nighters" for party. They are often deficient in rapid-eye movement (REM) sleep, and this can lead to dulled mental processing and confusion.

SELF-PERCEPTION AND SELF-CONCEPT. The young adult years are very important in the process of self-definition and self-perception. Individuals are at risk for problems associated with self-concept in all areas of life. Personal, social, and occupational evaluation processes are continuous processes.

ROLE RELATIONSHIPS. Problems in the area of role relationships are closely tied to self-concept problems. The young adult has many different roles and often experiences difficulty in defining and balancing roles, relationships, and responsibilities. Categories include academic and work-related roles, roles within the family (such as daughter, sister, or "peacekeeper"), extended "friend" family, and those roles related to career aspirations and vocational choices.

SEXUALITY AND REPRODUCTIVE SYSTEMS. Young adults are at high risk for problems of sexuality and the reproductive systems. Problems in this area may involve both physiologic and psychosocial problems (such as promiscuity, unwanted pregnancy, sexually transmitted diseases, or confusion).

STRESS AND COPING PATTERNS. Individuals at this age often experience rapid change in many areas of their lives, resulting in stress. Many have not developed good coping skills or have developed maladaptive or pathologic coping mechanisms, such as blaming others for problems or alcohol and drug abuse.

VALUES AND BELIEFS. The newly developed values and beliefs of young adults may be in conflict with those of others — peers, employers, professors — causing stress. This age group also may experience problems as they question their own values and beliefs.

Risks and problems experienced by this population include:

- academic and/or employment difficulties
- accidental injuries
- acquaintance rape
- anorexia or bulimia
- communication problems
- depression
- drug or alcohol abuse
- poverty
- pregnancy
- sexual experimentation
- sexually transmitted diseases
- suicide
- unemployment

WOMEN

"[A woman] will probably live seven to eight years longer than [her] male counterparts, but [she] will log more doctor visits, more disability days, higher rates of illness, and greater use of health services — even when the statisticians control for pregnancy-related conditions" (Gentry 1986, p.8).

Women in American society fulfill a variety of roles which interact to affect their health status in complex ways. The cultural, social, and biological differences between women and men intimately affect not only their actual health status, but their use and evaluation of health services as well.

Nurses, most of whom are women, are familiar with the variety of roles women play in our society. Many women feel overwhelmed by the complexity of their lives and from the demands that come from conflicting roles. Four of these roles have a significant effect on the ways in which women interact with the healthcare system (see *Figure 16*):

- woman as caretaker
- woman as consumer
- woman as worker
- woman as patient

FIGURE 16. WOMEN'S HEALTH-RELATED ROLES

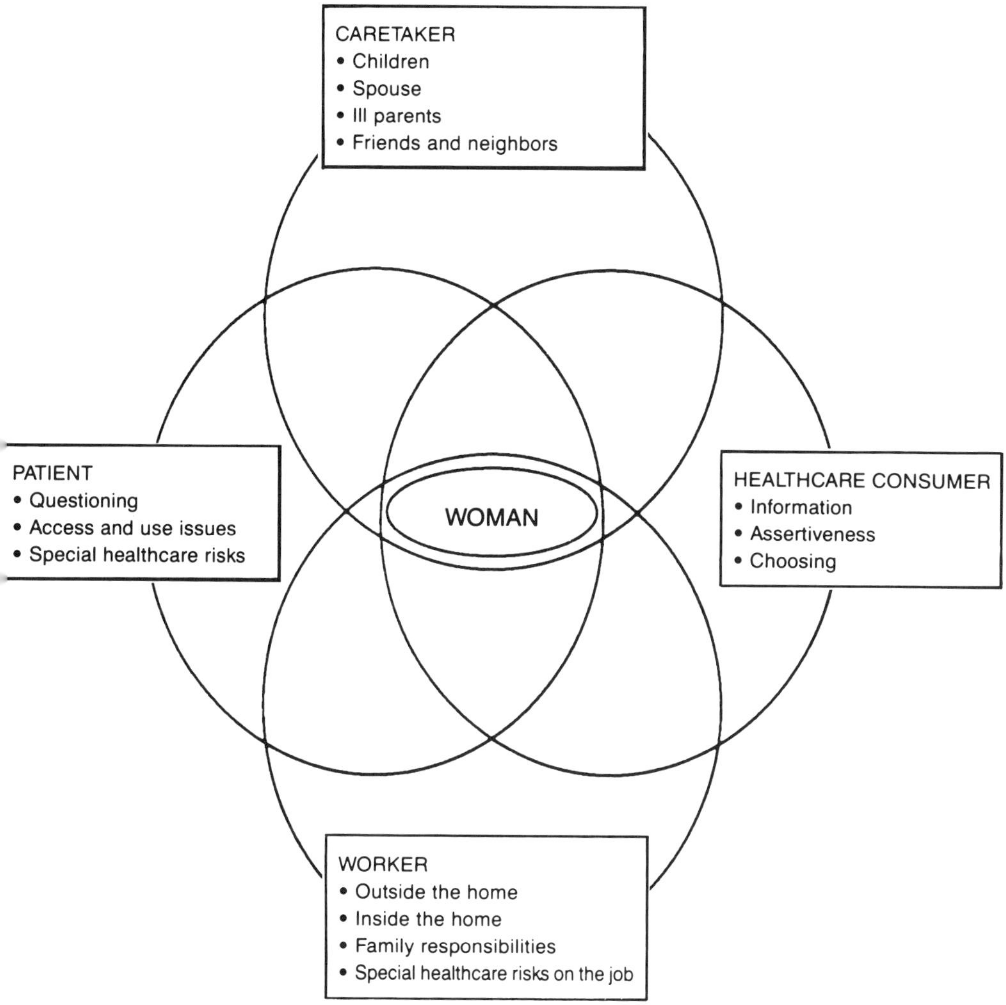

Women also face different risks to their health from those faced by men, due to a combination of biological and psychosocial factors.

WOMAN AS CARETAKER. The "typical" woman stands in the middle of a web of personal relationships — with a husband or boyfriend, children, siblings, parents, friends, neighbors, and coworkers. She is very likely to feel a sense of responsibility for the welfare of some or all of these persons. She is likely to become involved in physical and emotional caretaking activities which will place her in contact with healthcare providers, even when her own health status is not threatened. Mothers are the primary contact for pediatricians. Wives are typically very involved in accessing the healthcare system for their husbands and in managing their husbands' illnesses. Adult daughters and daughters-in-law care for their aging parents.

The caretaker role leads women to play another important role in the healthcare system: that of the primary healthcare consumer. In a study of telephone nursing services offered by a large midwestern health maintenance organization, it was found that females were the most frequent users of such services, with males as the most commonly reported patient/dependent (White 1989).

WOMAN AS CONSUMER. Women are the primary consumer decision makers for healthcare choices. They pick not only their own physicians, but also those consulted by their family members. Due to the fact that women are more likely to utilize healthcare services earlier in illness and more often than men, they become more "expert" in the use and evaluation of such services. Healthcare providers are beginning to recognize this fact, and are reorganizing and marketing services to attract women to their programs. Women are more likely to seek out information on health and illness and are more likely to pay attention to health information in the media (Weisman 1986). Studies have shown that at least 65 percent of all healthcare purchases are made by women (Alpern 1987).

WOMAN AS WORKER. More women than ever before are a part of the American work force. In 1987, 56 percent of women worked outside the home, and almost 52 percent of those with children under one year old worked outside the home (*Statistical Abstract* 1989). In addition, a woman's work does not end when she walks through the door at the end of the day; women are still primarily responsible for household and child-rearing tasks. These duties have been dubbed the woman's "second job" due to the fact that the amount of time needed to run a home and care for children is similar to a full-time job. And, because women have lower rates of employment, more intermittent employment, and lower earning power than men, they are at a disadvantage with regard to health insurance coverage, pension plans, and social security benefits. Economic disadvantage is well associated with risks to health, and there is no question that women are increasingly at risk for economic disadvantages: three-quarters of the poor in the United States are women and children (Gentry 1986).

WOMAN AS PATIENT. Women typically seek out healthcare services early in illness, when problems are less serious. "Women use health services more than men and are more likely than men to have a regular source of healthcare" (Weisman 1986, p.147). This is true even when all reproductive services are taken into account. Women ask more questions and are more likely to reveal their true concerns, whether these are physical or emotional. Studies have shown that they are interested not only in competent healthcare providers, but in empathetic care as well.

The risks to this population are centered in the following areas:

BIRTH CONTROL, PREGNANCY, AND CHILDBIRTH. Every birth-control method offers a different level of pregnancy risk and a different set of disadvantages for the couple. For a variety of reasons, unwanted pregnancies still account for over one-half of the pregnancies in this country. Women with unwanted pregnancies are at risk for emotional distress and a host of physical risks due to the possibility of poorer prenatal care. "Pregnancy care, [however], is one of the greatest medical success stories of this century" (Alexander 1986, p.10). There have been significant improvements in pregnancy outcome: the ability of medicine to deal with disorders during pregnancy, high-risk births, low-birth-weight infants, and premature births.

SMOKING AND LUNG CANCER. Lung cancer has surpassed breast cancer as the leading cause of cancer-related death for women as they have taken up smoking in greater and greater numbers. "The only portion of the population showing an increase in cigarette smoking is younger women" (Murray and Zentner 1985). Smoking is the most common form of drug dependency in our society, and it has a major impact on women's health.

ALCOHOLISM AND DRUG ABUSE. "Three and one-half million women are using alcohol inappropriately and may be classified as suffering from alcoholism" (Chatham 1986, p.17). A woman faces greater health consequences than a man from the consumption of identical amounts of alcohol, even when the women's smaller body is taken into consideration. "Alcoholic women die fifteen years earlier than nonalcoholic women and have a death ratio 50 to 100 percent higher than alcoholic men" (Gentry 1986, p.9). Alcoholic women are at higher risk for malnutrition, sleeping disorders, hormonal functioning problems, and many other disorders. Alcohol has a negative impact on every system within the body, and thus continued alcohol abuse exposes the woman to a wide variety of illness and disorders.

Women also face greater social stigma than men as a consequence of alcohol abuse (Gentry 1986). This makes it more difficult for women to seek help. In addition, alcohol use affects a woman's offspring; alcohol has a grave impact upon the developing fetus, and alcoholic mothers are less able to provide the care and nurturing necessary for the developing child. Fetal alcohol syndrome (FAS) is one of the three leading causes of birth defects associated with mental retardation (Brume 1986).

STRESS-RELATED DISORDERS. Due to the presence of greater numbers of women in the work force and those women's "second careers" as housewife and mother, women are at increased risk for stress-related disorders such as depression, headaches, sleeplessness, poor nutrition, and anxiety.

ECONOMIC RISKS. Poverty represents a serious risk to health. Women and their children currently make up approximately 75 percent of the nation's poor (Murray and Zentner 1985), and the conditions that have led to this situation continue to exist. Risks associated with poverty include malnutrition, poor health habits and medical care, unhealthful living conditions, high levels of stress, and low self-esteem.

OBESITY AND WEIGHT-LOSS DISORDERS. "Thin is in" and the pursuit of thinness poses health risks to women. Although younger women are more likely than adult women to develop anorexia and bulimia, excessive dieting can have very negative effects on a woman's health status and can even result in patterns of greater and greater weight gain. Obesity also creates risks: a greater chance of developing cardiovascular disease, certain kinds of cancer, and diabetes. The prevalence of obesity increases with age, as people become less physically active and their metabolism slows.

MENOPAUSE. The mean age of onset of the menopause in western societies is fifty-one years. Menopause brings with it not only biological changes but social changes as well; it is the end of the childbearing phase and all that it implies. The cessation of menses can signal the possible emergence of new health problems precipitated by estrogen loss. These include osteoporosis and vaginal dryness. Because the timing of menopause also coincides with other losses in life commonly experienced in middle age (such as children leaving home, parents become aging or dying, and major self-concept changes), psychosocial reactions to "menopause" may actually be reactions to the much larger issue of aging and mortality.

BREAST CANCER. The monthly breast self-exam is the easiest and most effective screening device with which women can reduce their risk of dying of breast cancer. It has been estimated that 95 percent of breast cancers are discovered by the woman herself. Women should also be encouraged to make use of mammographic services to supplement their own exams. Early detection greatly increases the odds of survival.

OSTEOPOROSIS. Osteopenia, the precursor of osteoporosis, is a detectable and potentially reversible disease. Some women are at higher risk for osteoporosis than others. Risk factors include family history, Caucasian or Asian racial background, childbearing and nursing patterns, nutritional status, activity level, and use of alcohol or cigarettes. The amount of bone loss can be measured by a diagnostic procedure called dual-photon absorpitometry.

HEART DISEASE. Although most people associate heart disease with men, heart disease is the leading killer of women in this country. In 1988, 240,000 women died of heart attack (as compared with 260,000 men). Because women have a sense of invulnerability to heart attack, many will ignore early signs and will not heed lifestyle warnings with regard to diet, stress, and exercise. Certain factors, such as smoking, obesity, high blood pressure, high blood cholesterol level, sedentary lifestyle, and selected personality characteristics (hostility, cynical mistrust of others, frequent angry outbursts), are thought to be associated with heart disease.

MEN

The "ideology of masculinity" prevents many men from expressing, and sometimes knowing, their true feelings (Julty 1979). In a healthcare situation, this can lead to men's downplaying the severity of their symptoms and not communicating their health concerns. Because the idealized image of the self-reliant male leads many men to wait to seek help until their conditions are serious, any male caller should be questioned thoroughly to make sure that all potentially important concerns are aired.

The "strong" male image belies many realities of men's lives: men live shorter lives, and are at higher risk for heart attacks and several types of cancer. They are more likely than women to be involved in violent crime (as perpetrators and victims), to be seriously mentally ill, and to be alcoholic or addicted to drugs. The special risks to this population are outlined below.

HEART DISEASE. Over one-half million people in the United States die every year of a heart attack. Men are more likely to die of heart attack than women, especially at younger ages. Factors that increase a man's risk for heart attack include cigarette smoking, high blood pressure, diabetes, inactivity, obesity, and a diet high in fat and cholesterol.

TESTICULAR CANCER. A self-diagnosis tool similar to the breast self-exam is the testicular self-exam, which should be used regularly by men to check for growths in the testes. Early detection and treatment substantially decrease mortality risk.

ALCOHOL AND TOBACCO ABUSE. An alcoholic is most likely to be a male over the age of thirty. Alcohol attacks every system in the body and leaves the alcoholic vulnerable to a variety of serious conditions, many of which are life-threatening. The regular and heavy use of alcohol further increases the man's risk for high blood pressure, which in turn increases his risk for heart attack. Tobacco use also raises the risk for heart disease, as well as for lung cancer.

HIGH BLOOD PRESSURE. Men face a higher risk for high blood pressure than do women. Because high blood pressure increases a man's risk for other serious problems and is not readily apparent without monitoring, blood pressure should be monitored on a regular basis, especially for those who are at a higher risk than the norm.

LUNG CANCER. More men than women die of lung cancer. It is the number one cancer killer of males, claiming nearly 85,000 lives each year. Smoking accounts for about 83 percent of lung cancer and 34 percent of all cancers in men. Those who smoke and work around toxic substances, such as asbestos, greatly increase their risk. The bottom-line advice for all patients is: *don't smoke*.

SENIORS

The elderly are growing, as a percentage of the overall United States population, at a brisk pace. Since 1900, the average life expectancy has increased by twenty-six years. There are more people over age sixty-five than under age twenty-five for the first time in history. People over age sixty-five represent 12 percent of the population and utilize 30 percent of all healthcare resources (Merck 1990).

Although the aging process begins to take effect after age thirty, individuals vary to the extent that they show the physical effects of growing older. With aging may come decreased vision, hearing, and taste. Many elderly persons lose significant pain response, placing these individuals at risk for injuries such as burns and frostbite. The elderly frequently present nonspecific or unexpected symptoms, which confuses diagnosis and may result in incorrect diagnosis and treatment.

Elderly patients visit physicians almost 50 percent more often than middle aged patients (Burton and Hazzard 1986). Many older adults experience multiple chronic conditions and have a need for frequent medical and nursing contact. One of the challenges posed by the elderly patient is separating new medical problems from manifestations of the aging process itself. Many treatable problems may be dismissed by vague assessments such as "you're just getting older," when in fact they should be evaluated and treated to improve the quality of the individual's life.

Older persons go through three stages of development in order to come to terms with life, and these may have an effect on health. First, employment and childcare roles are replaced with "new and meaningful" roles. Second, illness is transcended, as well as a preoccupation with the physical changes caused by aging, through the development of satisfying relationships and creative activities. Finally, satisfaction is achieved through contributions to others and society.

Women continue to live longer than men. At age eighty-five, the ratio of women to men is four to one. Therefore, in many ways, the care of the elderly is really the care of elderly women.

Like the other populations, this population carries its own special health risks:

LIVING ALONE. Among men and women over age sixty-five, 40 percent of women live alone, as compared with 15 percent of men (Banker, Burton, and Zieve 1986). Living alone can itself place the older adult at risk for a variety of ills: lack of support for daily living as well as during health crises, loneliness and depression, malnourishment (largely because of a lack of motivation to cook for one), and a reduced quality of life due to economic (one instead of two incomes) and social factors.

OSTEOPOROSIS. Osteoporosis, the weakening of bone due to calcium loss, affects 25 to 50 percent of women over the age of fifty. It involves the entire skeleton. At very advanced ages, osteoporosis is also found in males. Osteoarthritis is related to osteoporosis and involves degeneration of articular cartilage and hypertrophy of bone, causing pain, stiffness, and posture changes. Osteoporosis is considered a major precipitating cause of fractures in the elderly.

FALLS. Almost one-third of those over the age of sixty-five fall each year; one in forty will be hospitalized. Only about one-half of those hospitalized will still be alive just one year later. Falls are a major cause of disability and death in the elderly.

SLEEP DISORDERS. The "normal" eight-hour sleep cycle of the adult gradually changes and shortens to approximately six hours in the aged. Many elderly patients complain of insomnia, which may include problems falling asleep or staying asleep.

DEPRESSION. In a society that highly values its young and excludes or devalues its old, it is not unexpected that aging can represent a "depressing" prospect. Signs of depression may include somatic symptoms (such as fatigue, weight loss, and headaches); changes in sleeping patterns; memory disturbances or confusion; and feelings of sadness, loss, or hopelessness.

SUSCEPTIBILITY TO ILLNESS. Older adults are more susceptible to acute illness and should therefore avail themselves of immunizations against such illness as flu, pneumonia, hepatitis B, and tetanus.

BENIGN PROSTATE HYPERTROPHY (BPH). BPH is a common disease of the elderly male. It is the enlargement of the prostate gland, leading to symptoms such as urinary frequency and retention. The likelihood of a man's experiencing symptoms indicative of BPH are 50 percent at age fifty, rising to 90 percent at age ninety.

MALNUTRITION. Decreases in smell and taste sensation, combined with the loss of social cues for eating (for instance, family meals) can cause a decrease in food intake, leading to malnutrition. Anorexia can result from depression or illness (such as tuberculosis, cancer, lung disease, and heart disease).

URINARY INCONTINENCE. Incontinence is a problem for 15 to 30 percent of elderly women. The results of incontinence can be severe: social isolation, skin disorders, poor self-image, ruined sex lives, and other problems. It is a frequently stated reason for admission to a long-term-care facility. However, episodes of urinary incontinence can frequently be reduced through treatment. Living with this problem is not an inevitable consequence of aging.

CANCER. Lung cancer and breast cancer are the two biggest cancer killers of older women. Cancer of the cervix, while easily diagnosed via the Papanicolaou smear, remains a problem in the population of older women, who are, as a group, less likely to have regular tests performed.

The prognosis for those who discover breast cancer in its earliest stage is very good. Unfortunately, early detection methods (monthly breast self-exams and mammography) are underutilized, especially in the elderly population. Lung cancer has now become the number one cause of cancer death in women, surpassing even breast cancer.

HEART DISEASE. Cardiovascular disease accounted for over one-half of the deaths in 1988. Heart disease kills ten times more women than breast cancer.

IATROGENIC DISORDERS. Iatrogenic disorders are those induced by medical treatment. Nearly one-sixth of hospital admissions of patients over the age of seventy are related to adverse drug reactions (Banker, Burton, and Zieve 1986). Older patients experience drug-induced iatrogenic disorders for a variety of reasons:

- Aging affects metabolism and other factors that have an influence on drug tolerance.
- The elderly may show atypical presentations of disease, which can result in misdiagnosis or incorrect treatments (for example, wrong medication).
- Many elderly have multiple, chronic conditions, all of which may require medication. Different drugs may be prescribed by different practitioners, none of whom are communicating, and these medications may combine in ways detrimental to the individual.
- An elderly person may have problems following a treatment regimen, resulting in drug misuse.
- It has been estimated that over 70 percent of older patients are also using OTC drugs, many without their physician's knowledge.

CULTURAL ISSUES

> *It is more important to know what type of person has a disease than to know what type of disease a person has.*
>
> Sir William Osler

Culture shapes the way we view the world. It defines the meanings behind and the importance of all aspects of our lives, including our concepts of:

- family and friends
- work and leisure
- religion and spirituality
- health and illness

Our values and beliefs, the customs we follow, and the social structure within which we feel comfortable operating all grow out of our cultural heritage. Culture also shapes the ways in which we are willing and able to communicate with others.

Nurses need to be concerned with the cultural background of patients because it influences many everyday behaviors. Cultural identity shapes:

- the ways in which illness, physical hardship, pain, and death are experienced and handled
- the expectations patients bring into the nurse/patient relationship
- the types of care and treatment options sought, and what plans the patient will carry out
- lifestyle variables which influence health and vulnerability to disease

It is important that the nursing care offered to the patient be congruent with his or her values and beliefs. To provide care otherwise is likely to create a situation where the patient will withhold trust, information, and perhaps adherence to treatment plans.

In attempting to offer culturally congruent nursing care, nurses must be able to:

- identify their own cultural perspective so as to avoid biases toward a patient due to cultural identity
- identify the patient's cultural values which will critically influence his or her interactions with the healthcare "system" (including providers, environments, procedures)

- create a style of communicating with patients whose perspectives may be at odds with personal beliefs and values

One's cultural identity is not equal to one's ethnicity, although ethnicity and country of origin can provide clues to culturally based beliefs and values. Assessing ethnic group membership is not nearly as important for patient care as is assessing level of acculturation with Western culture and socioeconomic status (Leninger 1985).

Many illustrations of the relationship between culture and health care can be found in the real world; several examples follow:

- In studies assessing cultural differences in pain perception, significant differences were found in the ways in which different groups (White Anglo Saxon Protestants, Italians, Jews, and Irish) perceived, described, and dealt with pain (Rosenbaum 1989, and Moore and Dworkin 1988).
- Depression in the United States is perceived to be a pervasive problem; 15 percent of adults between the ages of eighteen and seventy-four suffer from symptoms of depression (Martinelli 1987). The same set of concerns may be perceived quite differently in many other countries in the world. For example, there is no word in colloquial Chinese to express depression. In China, mental illness is perceived as a political problem (Johnson 1986).
- In a study testing the knowledge and attitudes of three adolescent groups (Black, Latino, and White teenagers) about acquired immune deficiency syndrome (AIDS), substantial ethnic differences were found in knowledge about the transmission of AIDS (DiClemente 1988).
- Socioeconomic status is related to access to, use of, and comfort with healthcare organizations and professionals (Murray and Zentner 1985).

The United States healthcare system reflects the beliefs, values, and aspirations of the white, middle-class western culture that created it. In order to put aside biases when dealing with patients from other cultures, it is important to recognize just what those biases are. The American culture (Murray and Zentner 1985):

- sees illness as a challenge that can be defeated by the use of professional technological resources ("The War on Cancer")
- emphasizes that individuals should be productive and achieving; health is valued because it allows people to "get the job done"

- values technological solutions to human problems
- values change and expects people not only to cope well with change but to welcome it
- emphasizes the role of the individual (rather than the group), which leads to the valuing of assertive, independent healthcare consumers

It is important to examine one's own beliefs with regard to these views, as they influence one's language and manner when dealing with patients. In addition, nurses should identify the minority patient populations that are unique to their area of the country. Information should be compiled on the cultural belief systems of these populations, as well as vocabulary lists and other reference materials that will help deliver appropriate transcultural nursing care.

CHAPTER FIVE

TAKING THE TELEPHONE HISTORY

In obtaining the caller's chief complaint (CC), present illness (PI), and past history (PH), it is best to use open-ended or prompting questions. The need for information should be clearly explained to the caller. He or she should understand that when asked questions not directly related to his reason for the calling, needed information is being obtained to help determine the prime reason for the call. The details of medical, psychosocial, familial, and economic history are necessary to assess a problem accurately and to identify appropriate resources, and the caller must be made aware of this fact. All information must be synthesized to assess the patient's situation and to consider possible interventions.

THE CHIEF COMPLAINT (CC)

The "chief complaint" is the specific reason for the patient's call. It is important to determine the major problem facing the patient at this moment as well as its duration. (Why did the patient call, and why now?) The following steps should be taken by the nurse answering patient calls:

- Record the CC using the caller's own words (in quotation marks) whenever possible. It is important not to interpret or rephrase the patient's complaint.
- Attempt to have the patient identify the *major* problem (not a self-made medical diagnosis), even if he or she is experiencing several closely related complaints. These other problems will be addressed later in the call. If it is not possible to isolate one primary complaint, the CC will read "multiple complaints" and will provide a list of these complaints using the patient's own words.
- Begin the history taking with open-ended, neutral questions or statements, as free from confrontation, judgment, or misinterpretation as possible. "How may I help you?"; "Tell me about what is bothering you"; and "What problem led you to seek help?" are good ways to start. "What is your sickness?" implies that the patient is indeed sick. It is also important not to ask questions that are "multiple choice" in nature, as they can lead to confusion. For example, "Is the pain sharp, crushing, throbbing, cramping, burning, or like pins and needles?" is much more limiting than "Can you describe the pain?"
- Focus on one area at a time, allowing the caller time to tell the full story and facilitating descriptions whenever necessary with helping phrases such as "tell me more" or "go on." Clarifying information should be requested whenever there is uncertainty as to the precise meaning of statements.

- Do not translate the patient's complaint into a diagnosis. If the chief complaint was of passing black stools, it should be recorded as such, not as "gastrointestinal bleeding." "Chest pain" should not be translated into "angina pectoris."

The following are samples of desirable recordings of chief complaints because they are brief, specific, and to the point, In effect, they serve as introductions to the description of the present illness that will follow:

CC: "Terrible chest pain," 2-3 hours duration.
CC: "I've been throwing up," 8 hours duration.
CC: Cough, fever, insomnia of 4 days duration.

In general, the structure and process of the history via telephone do not differ markedly from an in-person interview. Because of the medium, however, the phone history requires specialized nursing skills to "fast forward" the process. The phone creates constraints which require special adaptation by the nurse to produce effective results. Just as during in-person interviews, identifying the real reason for the call often requires specialized interviewing skills and analysis; the true concern may not be the initially stated reason for the call.
The nurse should be able to identify: (1) the caller's chief concern; (2) the caller's perception of the severity of the problem; (3) the caller's level of concern about the problem; and (4) whether this level is appropriate, given the nurse's own assessment of the severity and urgency of the problem. For example, a woman calls to discuss her husband's strained finger (a recent basketball injury), and during the course of the conversation she also relates her concern about her husband's "breathing difficulties." She shares the fact that he must use four pillows underneath his head at night in order to breathe easily enough to sleep. The nurse in this scenario must address the breathing difficulties as a major concern while still dealing with the injured finger. Although the caller's identified problem was the spouse's sprained finger and did not include undue concern for the spouse's breathing difficulties, the nurse should communicate concern about the breathing difficulties to the caller. Callers often lack insight into their health problems and may perceive that they are more or less serious than they actually are. It is the nurse's responsibility to address these problems.

One approach the nurse can take to help define a caller's chief complaint is to address concerns as a loss or a potential loss. Many people will call because they are experiencing a loss or are afraid of experiencing a loss. These losses may include:

- loss of feeling "good" (healthy, happy)

- loss of normal functioning
- loss of activity due to health problems
- loss of ability to lead a normal life (work and play)
- loss of self-esteem and identity
- loss of ability to fulfill roles
- loss of independence
- loss of cognitive functions
- loss of opportunities (to achieve physical, psychological, or social goals)
- loss of a significant other, or any of the above losses relating to a significant other

PRESENT ILLNESS (PI)

A clearly worded narrative history of the present illness (shortened by necessity for phone histories) begins with the earliest onset of the complaint and describes the progression to the present. It is imperative to find out why it is that the caller called *now*. Thus "CC: Cough and fever, 3 days duration" should prompt an inquiry as to why the caller called today, not two days ago or yesterday. Did the cough become worse? Did the fever become worse? Did the cough change? Many valuable clues will be uncovered by obtaining the history of a complaint, from onset of symptoms to the present moment. Additionally, a fair amount of insight into the patient's personality and motivation may be uncovered by digging into details of the story. In the case of "CC: Cough and fever, 3 days duration," the nurse might uncover the fact that the patient's cough was no worse, but that he became afraid that he had pneumonia.

The following characteristics should be included in the description of the present illness:

- type
- location
- severity
- duration
- abruptness of onset
- precipitating or alleviating factors
- associated symptoms

Problems can then be classified according to functional health problems.

PAST HISTORY

An abbreviated past history, appropriate to the patient and problem, should be included in the history-taking process. Has the patient experienced this problem in the past? Does the patient have any chronic illnesses (such as diabetes, heart disease, cancer, or high blood pressure)? Has the patient been hospitalized?

Important information that is generally documented at the beginning of the history includes current medications, prescribed and over-the-counter. The nurse should ask specifically about some OTC medications (if pertinent) which many patients do not consider as medication (aspirin, for instance). Medications currently being taken should be recorded even if they do not relate to the stated reason for the call. Information concerning allergies, pregnancy (if female), and lifestyle factors (such as use of alcohol or drugs, exercise and sleep patterns, and stress) should also be obtained at the outset of the history, if at all relevant to the problem at hand.

REVIEW OF SYSTEMS (ROS)

A complete review of systems is inappropriate for the telephone history. However, the nurse should consider the patient's past health problems and the currently identified problem and perform a pertinent ROS of the relevant systems. For example, if the caller is a thirty-year-old woman with a concern of "stomach pain," the nurse should review the following systems (and others) should the need come to light during the proceeding sections of the history: gastrointestinal, genitourinary, gynecological, and psychosocial.

Although often thought of as a "wastebasket" portion of the patient history, the review of systems (ROS) is in fact a safety net for the nurse. Eliciting a pertinent ROS alerts the nurse to other related or coexisting problems, and allows a final check on the problem definition begun during the discussion of the present illness. Detailed questioning is essential for any additional symptom discovered. Significant negatives are important to document.

Many organizations have developed a standardized form for the ROS, thus minimizing the time it requires during a call. It should be remembered that there is no possibility of asking all possible questions of any given patient. Each nurse must develop a series of general, open-ended screening questions for each body system — for example, "Has there been any difficulty with hearing?"

Most patients, of course, will have had some history of at least minor problems which may be revealed during the ROS. The patient may not understand that in some instances seemingly minor problems may be significant in clarifying the story of the current problem. On the other hand, afflictions that are quite irritating to the patient, but unrelated, may shed no light on the immediate problem. How the nurse asks the questions is obviously of great importance and will vary with the nature of the complaint and with the individual patient.

Most nurses will need a partial or complete checklist to cover the patient's history thoroughly. There are multiple approaches for system review: head to toe, physical to social, or anatomical and functional, to name three. The section that follows contains a system review approach that includes some aspects of anatomical and functional approaches. The psychosocial system review is included early because some elements of psychosocial systems are important to review with each phone call. This list has been adapted for use by nurses on the phone. All portions of the ROS relevant to the chief complaint should be investigated and recorded in call documentation.

GENERAL. Overall state of health, fatigue, unexplained weight changes, exercise tolerance, fevers, frequent infections, ability to carry out activities of daily living, allergies, environmental factors, medications (prescribed and OTC).

PSYCHOSOCIAL SYSTEM. Cognitive abilities, response to problem, response to past care, cultural implications.

SOCIOLOGICAL STATUS. Family relationships, occupational history, economic status, educational level, patterns of health care.

INTEGUMENT. Sun exposure, past and current; tanning bed or parlor use; regular use of any skin creams, lotions, or cosmetics; eruptions, rashes, masses, pruritus; unusual pattern of hair loss; deformity or disorders of nails.

HEAD, EYES, EARS, NOSE, AND THROAT. Headaches; visual problems; smell; tongue or buccal sores, recurrent or chronic; nasal obstruction; epistaxis, difficulty in swallowing or speech, history of trauma. Glasses worn (if so, date of last refraction); cataracts, recent changes in vision. Hearing; ringing or buzzing in ears; environmental or industrial noise exposure; history of ear infections; ear discharge.

TEETH AND GUMS. Dental problems, chewing, fit of dentures (if present); bleeding or swelling of gums; dryness or excessive salivation; odors; pain. Frequency of and last professional cleaning.

RESPIRATORY. Wheezing; cough; hemoptysis; sputum production; shortness of breath at rest or on exertion; orthopnea; paroxysmal nocturnal dyspnea. Smoking history, date of last chest x-ray.

BREASTS. History of breast masses; performance of breast self-exam; nipple or breast skin changes; nipple discharge; pain or redness; mammography.

CARDIOVASCULAR. Chest pain; palpitations; fainting; heart murmur; leg or ankle edema; hypertension; claudication; varicose veins.

GASTROINTESTINAL. Appetite, dietary habits, food intolerance; bowel habits; jaundice; abdominal pain; indigestion; vomiting; hematemesis; bleeding; passing of tarry stools.

GENITOURINARY. Dysuria, frequency, urgency, hesitancy, nocturia, force of stream, bleeding; stones; venereal disease. History of urinary tract infections, renal or cystic calculi, or flank pain. History of sexually transmitted disease, discharge, or genital lesions. Sexual activity and level of satisfaction with it. For men: performance of regular testicular self-examination.

GYNECOLOGICAL. Menarche; catamenia, menorrhagia, metrorrhagia, dyspareunia, postcoital bleeding; type of contraception (if used), vaginal discharge; obstetrical history; date and results of last Pap smear; menopause and date.

MUSCULOSKELETAL. Weakness; neck, back or joint stiffness; pain or swelling; radicular pain; muscle cramps; arthritis; history of fractures; dislocations.

NEUROPSYCHIATRIC. *General*: syncope, seizures, vertigo, tremors, dizziness. *Intellect*: orientation to time, place and person, sensorium, memory. *Sensory*: paresthesia, hyperesthesia, hypesthesia. *Affect*: anxiety, nervousness, depression.

LYMPHATIC AND HEMATOLOGIC. Lymph node swellings; excessive bleeding or bruising; anemia; blood transfusions.

ENDOCRINE. Intolerant to weather changes; thyroid disorder; sugar in blood or urine; polydipsia, polyphagia, polyuria; excessive sweating.

NUTRITION. Eating schedule and balance in diet. Underweight, overweight, and any weight-altering behaviors (special diets and related issues).

MEDICATIONS AND SUBSTANCES THAT CAN ADVERSELY AFFECT FUNCTIONING.

- *Cognition and perception*:
  Alcohol
  Antibiotics
  Antiseizure medications
  Antidepressants
  Aspirins
  Tranquilizers
  Sedatives

- *Sleep and rest*:
  Alcohol
  Caffeine
  Sleep aids (OTC)
  Narcotics
  Antidepressants
  Amphetamines

- *Sexuality and reproductive function*:
  Alcohol
  Ametidine
  Antidepressants
  Antihistamines
  Antihypertensions
  Antispasmodics
  Barbiturates
  Caffeine
  Diuretics
  Narcotics
  Sedatives
  Tranquilizers

- *Elimination — bladder*:
  Antidepressants
  Antihistamines
  Antiparkinsonians
  Belladonna
  Phenothioziades
  Diuretics

- *Elimination — bowel*:
  Antacids
  Antibiotics
  Antidepressants
  Antihistamines
  Antiparkinsonians
  Belladonna
  Diuretics
  Phenothiozides
  Tranquilizers
  Narcotics

CHAPTER SIX

PERSONNEL CONSIDERATIONS

The most important aspect of a telephone nursing program is the nurses themselves: their skills, abilities, talents, expertise, and training. Proper recruitment, selection, training, supervision, evaluation, and rewards are critical for the success of a telephone nursing program. Many organizations have invested tens or hundreds of thousands of dollars in the quality of software and marketing programs utilized by their telephone nursing service without investing in the true backbone of the program: its nurses. Only they, through appropriate nursing practice, can accomplish the goals of telephone nursing: to provide continuing access to care in a manner consistent with the high standards set by the organization and the profession. Once practice standards are set, individual nurses and the program itself should be evaluated regularly to ensure that standards are upheld. (A sample peer evaluation form is provided as an appendix to this book. This can be used to help nurses evaluate each other as a part of internal evaluation and staff development efforts.

POSITION REQUIREMENTS

The telephone nurse systematically incorporates the steps of the nursing process: assessment, nursing diagnosis/problem definition, planning, implementation and evaluation. He or she provides access to health care and continuing care to individuals, families, and communities.

Nurses who work in telephone nursing must be educated and trained. Currently, centralized programs in nursing education do not address the special skills required for telephone nursing. Requirements for the telephone nurse who is responsible for clinical decisions include: the completion of a course of study in nursing leading to an associate degree, diploma, or baccalaureate degree in nursing, as well as passing scores on a state board examination for professional nursing. The baccalaureate degree in nursing is the preferred educational background for this position. Two years of ambulatory or hospital nursing experience are also desirable. Nurses who have emergency room experience and expertise usually have excellent backgrounds and preparation for telephone nursing.

The nurse must demonstrate clinical competence and decision making in nursing care via the telephone. This includes:

- triage
- case finding
- health information
- education

- resource identification
- consultation with and referral to physicians and other healthcare providers and services
- integration of these areas
- follow-along and follow-up care

STANDARDS AND PERFORMANCE CRITERIA

All activities associated with telephone nurse recruitment, selection, training, supervision, evaluation, compensation, and rewards flow from the creation of practice standards for telephone nursing. These standards form a basis for determining the quality of care which a telephone nurse provides. They define the nurse's obligation to provide and continually improve practice. They also allow for the definition of a rating system useful in evaluating individual performance.

Standards are useful to the organization in the following areas:

- *recruitment decisions* — who should be sought to fill a position
- *selection decisions* — who should be chosen from available candidates
- *training decisions* — how and what newly chosen telephone nurses should be taught
- *supervision decisions* — how telephone nurses should be supervised
- *evaluation and compensation decisions* — what aspects of telephone nursing practice are most important for effectiveness

Practice standards for telephone nurses should incorporate standards for each of four broad areas: (1) clinical practice, (2) education, (3) leadership, and (4) professionalism. The rating continuum outlined below allows for four different categories of performance evaluation for each of the four areas of telephone nursing practice. The "meets standards" rating identifies those who have demonstrated competent practice; "exceeds standards" identifies those who consistently excel; and "fails to meet standards" and "at times does not meet standards" identify those who do not demonstrate competent telephone nursing practice, either consistently or inconsistently. These standards reflect the consumer's criteria for quality as well as the expectations of the professional community and medical and nursing regulatory agencies.

CLINICAL PRACTICE

The standards for clinical practice are based on the nursing process. These are:

1. *Nursing assessment* is accomplished through interviewing. The nurse considers the problem using a holistic view of the patient and his or her unique characteristics and environment.
2. Problem identification (or nursing diagnosis) defines the impact of health problems affecting individuals and families so that appropriate information, education, and referral can be provided. The goal is also to help the patient and family cope with problems and situations. Nurses distinguish between normal and abnormal findings in order to identify patient capabilities and limitations.
3. Planning is the process of making decisions and setting goals with the patient and family. These must be acceptable to the nurse, patient, and pertinent others, including physicians and other healthcare professionals.
4. Implementation activities must include behavior that is:
   - caring (suggestions are made to make the patient comfortable);
   - curing (care is based on scientific principles, using the nursing process to identify and manage nursing diagnoses);
   - counseling (emotional, intellectual, and psychological support is provided, to include health promotion, patient education, and the full use of self in therapeutic relationships with patients);
   - facilitating (a liaison role provides for continuity of care between home, office, in-patient setting, and community).
5. *Evaluation* includes assessment of the outcomes and the patient's progress toward the achievement of goals or lack thereof. The nurse should direct the reassessment of goals and/or plans when evaluation necessitates.

The performance criteria for clinical practice are:

MEETS STANDARDS.

1. *Direct care*: Demonstrates clinical competence in providing care, via the phone, to patients and families in an established area of practice (centralized or decentralized, primary or specialty areas).
2. *Documentation*: Documents accurately and completely, and keeps statistics regarding telephone practice.
3. *Consultation/Collaboration*: Shares information with other members of the healthcare team. Makes appropriate requests for consultation and referrals. Identifies and wisely uses organizational and community resources. These include programmatic, personnel, informational, and financial resources.

EXCEED STANDARDS.

1. *Direct care*: Engages patients and families as active participants in their care. Maintains continuity of care through appropriate follow-up. Serves as a patient advocate.
2. *Documentation*: Documentation includes assessment, diagnosis, plans, and interventions.
3. *Consultation/Collaboration*: Shares information appropriately and seeks out others to assist in defining problems and recommending interventions.

EDUCATION

Education imparts knowledge and helps patients to develop skills, enhance decision making, and promote understanding. It includes interaction with the patient, family, and community, and may involve participation in formal and informal professional education. The standards for education are:

1. Teaches appropriate techniques or presents information necessary for health management.
2. Engages in ongoing evaluation of the effectiveness of teaching in terms of understanding and application.
3. Achieves patient goals as demonstrated by patient outcomes.
4. Develops new opportunities, tools, and methods of teaching appropriate for nursing via telephone.

The performance criteria for education are:

MEETS STANDARDS.

1. *Patient/Family/Community*: Identifies patient and family needs, and develops a plan for education and/or makes appropriate referrals. Teaches techniques or knowledge necessary for prevention, management, or rehabilitation.
2. *Professional*: Participates in educational programs in the clinic, hospital, extended-care facility, and community.

EXCEEDS STANDARDS.

1. *Patient/Family/Community*: Engages in the ongoing evaluation of teaching effectiveness in terms of patient understanding and adherence. Demonstrates achievement of teaching goals through patient outcomes. Develops new opportunities, tools, and methods of teaching.
2. *Professional*: Organizes educational programs in the clinic, hospital, extended-care facility, and community.

LEADERSHIP

Nursing leadership is the process through which the nurse affects the actions of others in goal determination and achievement. It includes decision making, communicating, influencing, facilitating, and problem solving. The telephone nurse:

1. Serves as a catalyst for improving standards of nursing practice.
2. Demonstrates leadership skills through the ability to set and attain goals.
3. Serves as a role model for professional telephone nursing conduct and practice.
4. Provides support to professional and technical staff.

The performance criteria for leadership are:

MEETS STANDARDS.

1. *Role modeling*: Serves as a role model in the enhancement of nursing practice and professional conduct. Demonstrates flexibility in performing additional responsibilities to contribute to the improvement of patient care.
2. *Goal determination/Achievement*: Formulates personal and professional goals which promote individual growth, utilizing appropriate resources. Integrates personal and professional goals with that of the medical group.
3. *Decision making/Problem solving*: Demonstrates ability to assess and solve problems. Serves as a member of a committee that enhances the quality of nursing care and the practice environment.
4. *Communication skills*: Develops positive communication skills with patients, families, coworkers, and physicians.

EXCEEDS STANDARDS.

1. *Role modeling*: Serves as a catalyst in improving standards of nursing practice. Plans with staff to implement needed changes. Demonstrates the ability to effect change in nursing practice. Develops methods for implementing and evaluating standards of care or works with others to develop such standards.
2. *Goal determination/Achievement*: Formulates and attains personal and professional goals which promote individual growth and advancement of nursing in the medical group or community, with minimal supervision. Creatively and independently formulates and attains personal and professional goals which promote individual growth and advancement of nursing.

3. *Decision making/Problem solving*: Anticipates problems and engages in sound problem-solving techniques. Serves as a member of a committee on healthcare decision making and policy in the organization or community.
4. *Communication skills*: Maximizes communication skills; involves patient for purposes of collaborative decision making, which results in increased self-care practice. Maintains open channels of communication; assists others in overcoming barriers of communication. Improves channels of communication and independently evaluates problem-solving activity among coworkers.

PROFESSIONALISM

Professionalism includes knowledge, self-direction, accountability, and the ability to use sound judgment in decision making. Professionalism in nursing involves a commitment to the improvement of human life and to the spirit of inquiry. The standards of professionalism for the telephone nurse are:

1. Demonstrates patient advocacy which ensures informed consent, including the areas of healthcare costs and research.
2. Maintains current clinical practice by selecting appropriate avenues for professional growth.
3. Utilizes and conducts research and inquiry appropriate to the clinical setting.
4. Remains accountable for the efficient use of time, material, and human resources.

The performance criteria for professionalism are:

MEETS STANDARDS.

1. *Patient advocacy*: Acts as a patient advocate by maintaining patient confidentiality; provides current information about health issues, diagnostic and therapeutic procedures, and prescribed medication and therapies.
2. *Professional growth*: Participates in professional conferences, workshops, and continuing education. Selects appropriate avenues for professional growth and attains at least the minimum number of contact hours per year required to maintain state licensure for professional nursing. Belongs to a professional organization.
3. *Research*: Utilizes clinical research to upgrade practice and improve patient care.
4. *Resource utilization*: Demonstrates efficient management of time and resources. Updates telephone nursing guidelines and

procedures. Adheres to organizational policies and nursing philosophies.

EXCEEDS STANDARDS.

1. *Patient advocacy*: Acts as a patient advocate by providing patients with informed-consent information regarding healthcare costs and patient rights. Participates in the development and implementation of services which identify healthcare options, risks, and benefits. Ensures patient participation in decision making with regard to services.
2. *Professional growth*: Selects appropriate avenues for professional growth beyond minimum requirements in area of practice. Relates learned information to the care of patients and families in the clinical and community setting. Develops and implements new cost-effective and high-quality services reflecting the "state of the art" in nursing practice.
3. *Research*: Participates in research which improves patient care. Acts as a coinvestigator or coauthor in compiling research results. Submits manuscripts for possible publication.
4. *Resource utilization*: Identifies methods to improve efficiency of time and resource management. Assists in the development of, or develops independently, methods to improve the efficiency of resource usage. May also independently implement and/or evaluate methods.

JOB DESCRIPTION

The job description is written to give a comprehensive and accurate portrait of the effective telephone nurse. It is the basis for developing standards of practice and performance review, as well as those standards needed to make hiring decisions.

An accurate, well-thought-out description enables the organization to undertake the appropriate recruitment, selection, and training activities prior to the nurse's actual starting date. It also ensures that the nurse adequately understands the parameters of the job, its responsibilities and accompanying expectations, prior to undertaking the commitment to accept the position. The description must define the scope of practice as well as the roles that the nurse must play during the course of his or her duties (medically dependent, interdependent, and independent). It should be based upon the respective state nurse practice acts and professional standards, organizational policies and procedures, and unit-specific policies and procedures.

The description should define and summarize the following aspects of the telephone nursing position:

- purpose of the telephone nurse
- level of responsibility given to the telephone nurse
- degree of supervision given the telephone nurse
- expectations associated with the position
- specific responsibilities
- required knowledge, skills, educational attainments, and experiences needed to fulfill position's duties
- description of working conditions

The following "generic" telephone nursing job description can be easily adapted to most organizations and specialty units.

GENERAL SUMMARY. The telephone nurse practices nursing via the telephone utilizing the nursing process and physician- and organization-approved telephone nursing guidelines. The functions of this position include triage, case finding, providing information and education, identifying resources, consultation and referral, and appropriate follow-up activities. All duties and responsibilities must be accomplished within the guidelines for the unit, department, and organization and in compliance with state laws and medical and nursing standards of care. Each telephone nurse reports to (*title of supervisor*).

PRINCIPAL DUTIES AND RESPONSIBILITIES.

1. The telephone nurse conducts phone interviews and assessments of patients with real or potential, acute and/or chronic health problems. These may include physical, psychosocial, or cognitive problems.
2. The telephone nurse explains medical terms and procedures.
3. The telephone nurse provides information regarding prescribed medications and therapies, utilizing appropriate physician consultation.
4. The telephone nurse identifies patient, family, physician, organization, and community resources and assists patients in gaining access to these resources.
5. The telephone nurse refers patients to physicians, other health team members, and programs.
6. The telephone nurse develops and implements follow-up procedures.
7. The telephone nurse acts as a liaison between physician, office, in-patient settings, home and community.
8. The telephone nurse records, communicates, and documents data from phone calls to ensure a high quality of care, effective

continuity of care and prudent risk management for the organization.

9. The telephone nurse maintains and enhances an up-to-date level of knowledge regarding professional telephone nursing practice.

REQUIREMENTS.

1. Licensed professional nurse.
2. Two years related nursing experience.
3. Knowledge of appropriate scope of nursing practice via the phone and ability to articulate this scope of practice.
4. Professional knowledge and clinical nursing skills in the following areas:
   - all steps of the nursing process
   - medical diagnoses
   - health sciences
   - pharmacology
   - emergencies
   - problem-oriented medical records and SOAP charting procedures
5. High level of creative problem-solving skills. Priority-setting skills. Ability to use these skills in environments where the nature and volume of calls is unpredictable.
6. Interpersonal skills necessary to provide care, instruction, and persuasion by phone and to collaborate with other health team members.
7. Physical ability to sit for extended periods of time. Mental attentiveness and skills necessary to address a variety of problems and callers within short periods of time.

WORKING CONDITIONS. The telephone nurse works in an environment where there may be frequent interruptions and where demands often seem to exceed the supply of time. At other times, utilization may be low, requiring the nurse to be self-motivated to develop guidelines and procedures for the department.

CHAPTER SEVEN

PUTTING IT ALL TOGETHER

The best approach for the assessment and management of the patient is the care of a competent nurse who looks upon the patient as a person and who deals with that person's problem in a holistic framework. If a structured, holistic approach to handling calls is incorporated into nursing practice, it will naturally lead to asking the right questions and getting the right answers for a thorough assessment.

Because health is much more than simply the absence of disease, and illness is an interaction of one or more problems in a specific person, assessment of any person's health status requires a synthesis of information about the whole person: his or her problems, personal resources, and the nature of the illness. Absence of adequate information about any of these elements leads to less than optimum patient care.

Gaining information about the person is dependent upon obtaining an adequate health history with accurate information about past medical history, family history, and personal and social history. An important step in total assessment is the establishment of a nursing diagnosis, or, in terms of the problem-oriented approach, the assessment of the patient's problem.

The establishment of a correct problem definition depends upon two major processes: the collection of information (subjective and objective) from the patient and the analysis of that information. No proper or complete analysis can be made if the data base is inadequate or in error. Information must be collected as systematically and as thoroughly as possible, given the limitations of the telephone. The nurse must be able to perform this type of interview and analysis quickly to determine the urgency and severity of the caller's problem, and to engage in case finding, resource identification, and appropriate follow-up and referrals. Knowing one's limitations and knowing when referral is in order are critical aspects of the process of telephone nursing. An approach to quick assessment is outlined in *Figure 17*.

The development of rapport and trust during a relatively short telephone interaction with the patient is a major goal in the assessment process. Rapport and trust are also significant factors in the management of the patient's problems. The interview is a part of the therapeutic process as well; it helps to establish a therapeutic relationship, not only with the individual nurse but with the healthcare "system" as well. Positive and helpful contact with the patient plays a role in reducing the patient's anxiety and uncertainty.

FIGURE 17.
TELEPHONE NURSING QUICK ASSESSMENT PROCESS

1. WHO IS THE CALLER?
   All of the information that has been gathered about the caller should be summarized: allergies, medications, past health problems, family situation (people, finances, environment), employment.

2. WHAT IS THE STATED CONCERN OR QUESTION?
   This includes information provided by the caller as well as the symptoms described.

3. WHAT ARE THE RISKS?
   Based on the answers to the first two questions, risks related to age, sex, culture, physical, or psychosocial considerations can be ascertained.

4. TRIAGE: WHAT ARE THE WORST THINGS THAT COULD BE HAPPENING IN THIS SITUATION?
   The answer to this question is determined based on the information provided by the answers to the first three questions.

5. WHAT ARE THE MOST IMPORTANT QUESTIONS TO ASK?
   The most important questions should be asked first. For example, if a person calls complaining of a cough, and the nurse finds out there is respiratory distress, he or she can proceed directly to obtaining emergency assistance for the caller.

6. IS THE PROBLEM NONURGENT?
   If the nurse determines the problem is not urgent and/or severe, the structured assessment process (including appropriate review of systems) is completed based on information that is both subjective (what the caller says) and objective (what the nurse hears).

7. WHAT ARE THE PROBLEMS AND THE RESOURCES?
   A list of problems and available resources should be developed, including the patient, family, healthcare providers, community and national organizations.

8. WHAT IS THE TIME FACTOR?
   The time of day, the day of the week, the season of the year all may be important considerations.

9. WHAT IS THE PLAN?
   A plan should be developed to include goals, timeliness, and evaluation criteria ("The caller will do . . ." and "The telephone nurse will do . . .").

10. WHAT INFORMATION SHOULD BE DOCUMENTED?
    All important information gathered from questions one to nine should be documented using SOAP notes.

DOCUMENTATION

The liability assumed by the practitioner after telephone contact is much the same as that assumed after physical contact (J.L.Brown 1980). The nurse is legally responsible for the care and advice given over the phone and should behave accordingly.

A written record of the content of all patient calls must be kept. While many telephone nursing practices allow a simple "log" system to be used, such practices serve neither the informational nor the legal needs of the nurse. Informational needs include the necessity of assessment, problem definition (nursing diagnosis), and planning information for sharing with future caregivers, ideally as a part of the patient's file. Legal needs include the necessity of being able to demonstrate accurately the specific information given by the caller and the advice given to the patient by the nurse. Documentation is not the best defense — it is the *only* defense. The medical record is the first, and probably the most important evidence a plaintiff's attorney will examine to establish a claim of negligence against the nurse (J.L.Brown 1980).

Actual information in the written record should include:

1. Information gathered during assessment (subjective history and objective findings per hearing sense), especially that information which leads to the problem definition and nursing assessment (severity and urgency).
2. The nursing diagnosis and nursing plan, as given to the caller.
3. Any advice, instruction, or other information given to the caller.
4. The caller's response: agreement or disagreement with advice and instruction or other information given by the nurse. (If the nurse recommends that the caller go to emergency room and the caller refuses, that refusal should be noted in the record.)
5. Any consultation and recommendations made by other practitioners.
6. Planned follow-up activities.

(A sample of a complete documentation form is provided as an appendix to this book.)

PRACTICE STANDARDS

The telephone nurse should operate within a set of practice standards which describe expected nursing behaviors and allow an assessment of the quality of care given. Some of these grow out of the standards set for the individual nurse (see the American Nurses' Association and the International Council of Nurses codes for nurses included in the appendixes); others are unique to a specific institution or program; and others serve as a quality-control mechanism for the entire telephone nursing program. Once practice standards are set, internal mechanisms for practice evaluation should be created and used.

Consultation and referral is one area that calls for practice standards. The telephone nurse, due to the limitations of the telephone and both the nurse's and the institution's legal liability for care, should always consult with colleagues or refer the caller to a physician if there are any doubts about his or her ability to assess, define problems, or advise the patient.

Names, addresses, telephone numbers, and other information about available resources should be organized and readily available to the telephone nurse via rolodex or software. Because the goal is to provide information to the caller while minimizing waiting time, this resource information should be as comprehensive as possible and should be located in close proximity to the nurse. A list of important resources is provided in Figure 18.

FIGURE 18. IMPORTANT RESOURCES

- **Protocols and telephone nursing guidelines**
- **Emergency criteria (available from the American Hospital Association)**
- **Information on medication (*Physicians' Desk Reference*)**
- **Reference on communicable diseases**
- **Reference on diagnostic and laboratory tests**
- **Referral sources: physicians and organizations (community and national)**
- **Emergency phone numbers**
- **Community resources**

LEGAL ISSUES

Nursing liability is an area of growing concern. Nurses have a duty to provide competent care which includes (McDonough 1990):

- identifying and intervening in situations in which care by others may jeopardize the patient
- not accepting assignments where a patient's needs are beyond the nurse's ability
- making judgments to carry out or question physician orders
- providing the physician with vital information concerning the patient

It is important to recognize and emphasize that telephone nurses do not engage in medical diagnosis. Although many physicians treat patients over the phone, they are not immune to the legal dangers of diagnosing a patient who is not examined: "It only takes one lawsuit for a bad result to wipe out years of cost effectiveness. You can't defend your diagnosis if you did not examine the patient. The law does allow mistakes in judgment if you based your decision on a competent evaluation of the situation" (Fish and Ehrhardt 1989, p.13).

The telephone nurse only engages in approved nursing behaviors, using the nursing process and the organization's approved telephone nursing guidelines as a tool. Nurses must be very careful that they do not engage in activities defined as medical diagnosis. The patient must be informed, as a normal part of every call, that the nurse's role is to assess severity and urgency, provide health information, and facilitate access to the appropriate level of care, whether through physicians or other healthcare providers and resources. The nurse helps the patient make informed decisions about his or her own health care and the options available to facilitate that care. If, as a part of the assessment process, the nurse comes to the conclusion that a patient needs to be seen by a physician, it is the nurse's responsibility to facilitate the patient's referral to the physician or emergency department.

Negligent conduct on the part of a nurse is a basis for malpractice litigation. The patient or relative must provide evidence about four issues: (1) duty, (2) breach of duty, (3) cause and effect, and (4) harm or injury (American Nurses' Association 1989).

DUTY. The nurse must protect the client against unreasonable risks by adhering to a certain code of conduct (for example, the American Nurses' Association standards).

BREACH OF DUTY. Breach of duty is most often determined by examining the documentation by the nurse.

CAUSE AND EFFECT. Cause and effect is a relationship between the nurse's conduct and an alleged injury.

HARM OR INJURY. There must be actual injury (physical or psychological) and loss, which can include economic loss, experienced by the patient.

Nurses are expected by the courts to exercise judgment. This involves interpreting signs and symptoms (severity and urgency), judging how to treat them (nursing diagnosis), and making appropriate referrals.

In short, telephone nursing involves responsibility for the quality of care provided and accountability. Nurses must accept that they are always accountable for their actions. Accountability implies duty and that a reasonable standard of care will be taken in the exercise of that duty. In the event a patient is harmed, nursing accountability becomes a measure of legal liability (Murchison et al 1978). Rather than fear legal responsibility, nurses should prepare for it by being well aware of the legal aspects of telephone nursing (McGear and Simms 1988).

Prevention tips for the most frequent allegations against nurses are provided in *Figure 19*. Nurses should adapt this list to their practice on the telephone.

GUIDELINES FOR PRACTICE

The following are general guidelines for telephone nursing practice:

1. Don't place a caller on hold until you know that his or her problem is not an emergency.
2. Your primary role at the beginning of the call (assessment phase), and your most valuable skill, is listening. Remember, you can only use the information you obtain through listening! You have no other senses on which you can rely. Ask open-ended questions, which serve not only to elicit information, but to reassure the patient:
   "Tell me more about it."
   "Anything else?"
3. Talk directly to the caller whenever possible, as others may not describe the problem accurately. If the caller cannot speak directly with you (due to hearing difficulty, language barrier, or other similar problem) advise the caller to come in. By the same token, if the

FIGURE 19. MOST FREQUENT ALLEGATIONS AGAINST NURSES AND PREVENTION TIPS

ALLEGATION	PREVENTION TIPS
FAILURE TO ENSURE PATIENT SAFETY	• Monitor patient in timely manner.* • Provide assistance for patients who require it when they need to use the lavatory or shower. • Keep bedrails raised for patients who are medicated or confused. • Use restraints appropriately.
IMPROPER TREATMENT OR PERFORMANCE OF TREATMENT	• Question treatments you believe are improper.* • Use proper techniques when performing procedures. • Follow hospital procedures when performing treatments. • Seek consultation for treatments beyond your abilities.* • Update your clinical skills through continuing education classes.*
FAILURE TO MONITOR AND REPORT	• Follow physician's orders regarding monitoring of patient.* • Report any requested information or significant changes in a patient's condition.* • Perform appropriate and timely nursing assessments.*
MEDICATION ERRORS AND REACTIONS	• Verify any questionable medical orders.* • Verify patient's name before administering medication.* • Listen to patient's objections regarding medication.* • Refer to *Physicians' Desk Reference* for any questions on appropriate dosages, side effects, and reactions.*
FAILURE TO FOLLOW HOSPITAL PROCEDURE	• Know your hospital's procedures.* • If you must deviate from a procedure, discuss the incident with your supervisor and decide the appropriate action.* • Advise the appropriate person of any procedures which need to be revised.*

*Special relevance for ambulatory care and telephone nurses

FIGURE 19. (continued)
OTHER COMMON ISSUES IN LAWSUITS

ISSUE	PREVENTION TIPS
DOCUMENTATION*	• Document significant information about your patients objectively and factually. • Be time-specific about the information, such as when you performed actions, made observations, or performed assessments. • Document legibly, spell correctly, and use only hospital-approved abbreviations.
EQUIPMENT USE	• Learn how to operate equipment in a safe and appropriate manner. • In teaching patients to use equipment, follow a predetermined procedure. • Provide home-care patients with the number of a 24-hour backup hospital or home-care service in case of emergency. • Have patients demonstrate their competence with equipment before allowing them to use it.
ADVERSE INCIDENTS*	• When adverse incidents occur, complete the appropriate documentation and report the incident to the designated individual. • Don't assume, voice, or record any blame for the incident.
PATIENTS WITH HUMAN IMMUNO-DEFICIENCY VIRUS (HIV)	• Be conscious of actions which could result in lawsuit: —discrimination in treatment —nosocomial (in-hospital) transmission of the virus —breach of confidentiality* —participation in testing a patient for HIV without first obtaining informed consent • Follow hospital procedures for care of patients with infectious diseases.

*Special relevance for ambulatory care and telephone nurses

(American Nurses' Association 1989)

subject of the call is too young to talk on the phone, and there is uncertainty regarding the problem, suggest a visit. This is especially true for infants.

4. Do not express surprise or judgment at the caller's statements.
5. Always express interest and concern for the caller's problems.
6. Remember that there is no adequate way to measure pain. It is important that the caller's description, rather than your interpretation, be recorded in call documentation. Always remember that the patient's perception is his or her reality.
7. Try to like your patient. It will make it easier to elicit information as your tone of voice and degree of attentiveness will put the caller at ease.
8. Don't believe everything you hear. Patients forget. Also, they may deliberately suppress information (often because of fear), they may unconsciously repress information, and they may falsify statements.
9. Avoid too many "why" questions. They are often challenges to the patient's competence. "Why did you stop taking your medication?" can lead to confrontation and hostility, whereas more neutral and open-ended expressions, such as "Tell me more about your reasons for not using the medication," may maintain rapport and obtain information.
10. Identify and remove barriers to communication between you and the caller.
11. Do not express judgment about the previous course of treatment given the patient by other practitioners. It is a safe assumption that neither you nor the patient has adequate information to make such judgments hastily.
12. Be certain that words used by you and the patient have the same meaning. Nurses know that all "swellings" are not cancers, but does the patient? Use medical jargon carefully to avoid misunderstandings. Be sure that the patient understands your language and questions clearly or his answers may be inaccurate.
13. Be as quantitative as possible. "At 2:00 p.m. yesterday, about a half hour after eating a large meal, Mrs. X vomited several quarts of partly digested food" is a quantitative and informative statement.
14. Keep in mind the patient's reason for seeking professional help. If he or she calls for treatment for a cold, don't forget this complaint as you get involved in other (perhaps more serious) aspects of the patient's problems.
15. Remember that you are the nurse and, therefore, the guide in the nurse/patient relationship. It is your responsibility to create a positive atmosphere in which you and the caller can work together to solve the problem.
16. Give specific instructions and try to verify the caller's understanding of those instructions. Discuss expectations ("If you still feel

nauseous in eight hours, call me back") as well as how to obtain care.

17. Have the caller repeat your instructions so that you are sure he or she understands them. Elicit the caller's degree of comfort with the interaction: "How does that sound to you?"
18. Respond to any anxiety exhibited by the caller. Do not assume that an objectively "minor" problem seems minor to the caller! If the caller remains anxious even after your attempts to calm him or her, advise the caller to come in. On the other hand, if the caller does not perceive a problem to be serious when you feel he or she is at risk, use persuasion and elicit physician assistance to facilitate appropriate care.
19. Your words and manner should reassure the caller that his or her concerns are being taken seriously.
20. If you feel unsure about your ability to assess the caller accurately (for whatever reason), refer the patient to a physician.
21. Allow the caller to respond to your assessment. You must create an "environment" within the call that allows the caller to correct your assessment or disagree if necessary. If the caller is not comfortable with either your assessment or your advice, suggest that the caller come in.
22. *Document* the call. From both quality assurance and legal perspectives, accurate, SOAP-formatted documentation is critical. "If it isn't documented, it didn't happen."
23. Provide the caller with information concerning immediate access to care: "A physician is available twenty-four hours a day in the emergency room."

This book expresses a philosophy and approach that can serve as a guide throughout the professional life of a nurse. Good nursing via the telephone can truly provide significant benefits for all involved — nurses, physicians, organizations, and most importantly, patients and the community — and ultimately lead to the improved efficiency and effectiveness of health care.

APPENDICES

APPENDIX A

AMERICAN NURSES' ASSOCIATION CODE FOR NURSES

INTRODUCTION

The development of a code of ethics is an essential characteristic of a profession and provides one means for the exercise of professional self-regulation. A code indicates a profession's acceptance of the responsibility and trust with which it has been invested by society. Upon entering the profession of nursing, each person inherits a measure of the responsibility and trust that has accrued to nursing over the years and the corresponding obligation to adhere to the profession's code of conduct and relationships for ethical practice.

The Code for Nurses, adopted by the American Nurses' Association (ANA) in 1950 and periodically revised, serves to inform both the nurse and society of the profession's expectations and requirements in ethical matters. The Code and the Interpretive Statements together provide a framework for the nurse to make ethical decisions and discharge responsibilities to the public, to other members of the health team, and to the profession. While it is impossible to anticipate in a code every type of situation that may be encountered in professional practice, the direction and suggestions provided here are widely applicable.

The Code for Nurses and the Interpretive Statements are both directed toward present-day practice. Previous Codes have been more prescriptive, identifying codes of both personal and professional behavior, describing appropriate relationships with physicians and other health professionals, and identifying certain responsibilities of the nurse as a citizen, an employee, and a person. The present Code, while remaining prescriptive, depends more on the nurse's accountability to the client, and, in that sense, represents a change to an ethical code.

The requirements of the Code may often exceed, but are never less than those of the law. While violations of the law may subject the nurse to civil or criminal liability, the constituent associations may reprimand, censure, suspend, or expel ANA members from the Association for violations of the Code. The possible loss of the respect and confidence of society and one's colleagues are serious sanctions which may result from violations of the Code. Each nurse has a personal obligation to uphold and adhere to the Code and to insure that nursing colleagues do likewise. Guidance and assistance in implementing the Code in local situations may be obtained from the American Nurses' Association or its state constituents.

PREAMBLE

The Code for Nurses is based on belief about the nature of individuals, nursing, health, and society. Recipients and providers of nursing services are viewed as individuals and groups who possess basic rights and responsibilities, and whose values and circumstances command respect at all times. Nursing encompasses the promotion and restoration of health, the prevention of illness, and the alleviation of suffering. The statements of the Code and their interpretation provide guidance for conduct and relationships in carrying out nursing responsibilities consistent with the ethical obligations of the profession and quality in nursing care.

CODE FOR NURSES

1. The nurse provides services with respect for human dignity and the uniqueness of the client unrestricted by considerations of social or economic status, personal attributes, or the nature of health problems.

2. The nurse safeguards the client's right to privacy by judiciously protecting information of a confidential nature.

3. The nurse acts to safeguard the client and the public when health care and safety are affected by the incompetent, unethical, or illegal practice of any person.

4. The nurse assumes responsibility and accountability for individual nursing judgments and actions.

5. The nurse maintains competence in nursing.

6. The nurse exercises informed judgment and uses individual competence and qualifications as criteria in seeking consultation, accepting responsibilities, and delegating nursing activities to others.

7. The nurse participates in activities that contribute to the ongoing development of the profession's body of knowledge.

8. The nurse participates in the profession's efforts to implement and improve standards of nursing.

9. The nurse participates in the profession's efforts to establish and maintain conditions of employment conducive to high quality nursing care.

10. The nurse participates in the profession's effort to protect the public from misinformation and misrepresentation and to maintain the integrity of nursing.

11. The nurse collaborates with members of the health professions and other citizens in promoting community and national efforts to meet the health needs of the public.

APPENDIX B

INTERNATIONAL COUNCIL OF NURSES CODE FOR NURSES

The fundamental responsibility of the nurse is fourfold: to promote health, to prevent illness, to restore health, and to alleviate suffering.

The need for nursing is universal. Inherent in nursing is respect for life, dignity, and rights of man. It is unrestricted by considerations of nationality, race, creed, color, age, sex, politics, or social status.

Nurses render health services to the individual, the family and the community and coordinate their services with those of related groups.

NURSES AND PEOPLE

The nurse's primary responsibility is to those people who require nursing care.

The nurse, in providing care, promotes an environment in which the values, customs, and spiritual beliefs of the individual are respected.

The nurse holds in confidence personal information and uses judgment in sharing this information.

NURSES AND PRACTICE

The nurse carries personal responsibility for nursing practice and for maintaining competence by continual learning.

The nurse maintains the highest standards of nursing care possible within the reality of a specific situation.

The nurse uses judgment in relation to individual competence when accepting and delegating responsibilities.

The nurse when acting in a professional capacity should at all times maintain standards of personal conduct which reflect credit upon the profession.

NURSES AND COWORKERS

The nurse sustains a cooperative relationship with coworkers in nursing and other fields.

The nurse takes appropriate action to safeguard the individual when his or her care is endangered by a coworker or any other person.

NURSES AND THE PROFESSION

The nurse plays a major role in determining and implementing desirable standards of nursing practice and nursing education.

The nurse is active in developing a core of professional knowledge.

The nurse, acting through the professional organization, participates in establishing and maintaining equitable social and economic working conditions in nursing.

APPENDIX C

NURSE ON CALL® TELEPHONE NURSING TRAINING PROGRAM COURSE OBJECTIVES

The NURSE ON CALL Telephone Nursing Training Program uses lecture, audiovisual materials, and exercises to communicate the essential characteristics of telephone nursing and the role of the telephone nurse.

The objectives for each nurse enrolled in this course are as follows:

- Can describe the roles of professional nurses in telephone nursing:

    1. the role of patient advocate
    2. the medically dependent role of the nurse
    3. the interdependent role of the nurse
    4. the independent role of the nurse

- Can describe the benefits of telephone nursing to callers, nurses, and healthcare organizations

- Can describe and demonstrate the use of the nursing process in telephone nursing

- Can identify the differences between telephone nursing and traditional ambulatory-care nursing

- Can describe concepts of nursing and health and their implications to nursing practice

- Can identify risk factors within groups in the patient population

- Can describe and demonstrate active listening and other verbal communication skills necessary to assess patients accurately

- Can describe ethical and legal issues relevant to the practice of telephone nursing

- Can identify emergencies, "red flags," and urgent problems in all functional areas and systems — physical, psychosocial, and environmental

- Can demonstrate knowledge and utilization of appropriate resources which can be used to benefit patients

- Can demonstrate the synthesis of the above and can integrate new knowledge and skills into telephone nursing practice.

APPENDIX D

TELEPHONE NURSING PROGRAM SAMPLE DOCUMENTATION FORM

The following form is used by one Nurse on Call site. In the form, a number of objectives are met through the recording of the following types of information:

- basic patient information and history
- descriptions of recommendations given (including referrals)
- follow-up plans
- demographic information helpful to planners and marketers

In addition, space is devoted to SOAP notes to ensure that the nurse is documenting relevant clinical information. The clinical and managerial information contained in this form can also be documented on computerized tracking software available from Nurse on Call.

DATE ____________________ HOW HEARD: ☐ RADIO ☐ PRINT AD
TIME ____________________ ☐ MD OFFICE ☐ YELLOW PAGES
TIME RETURNED _________ ☐ BROCHURE ☐ ____________________

PATIENT INFORMATION

PATIENT NAME ______________________________ AGE ________ SEX: ☐ M ☐ F
PHONE: ______________________ (home) ______________________ (work)
ADDRESS ________________ CITY ________________ STATE ________ ZIP ________
CALLER NAME (if different) ______________________________
RELATIONSHIP ____________________ REASON FOR CALL ____________________

PATIENT HISTORY

ALLERGIES ______________________________
CHRONIC DISEASE ______________________________
☐ PREGNANT? ☐ MEDICATIONS? ______________________________
CURRENT PHYSICIAN ______________________________ MD# ______________

CHIEF COMPLAINT/REASON FOR CALL
(SOAP notes)

____
____
____
____
____
____
____
____
____
____
____

RECOMMENDATIONS

SIGNS/SYMPTOMS TO OBSERVE ______________________________
____
HOME TREATMENT/TEACHING (diet, activity, etc.) ______________________________
____
CALLER'S RESPONSE ______________________________
____

FOLLOW-UP
(Note time and/or date after each item checked)

☐ ER REFERRAL ____________________ CONTACT PERSON ____________________
☐ HOME HEALTH REFERRAL ____________ CONTACT PERSON ____________________
☐ ER PHYSICIAN NOTIFIED ____________ ☐ CLIENT CALL BACK ______________
☐ CLIENT TO CALL MD ______________ ☐ NOC TO CALL MD ______________
☐ NOC TO CALL ____________________ ☐ OTHER DATE ____________________

☐ PLACE IN MEDICAL RECORDS ☐ HOLD IN OFFICE (release date __________)

APPENDIX E

NURSING ASSESSMENT WORKSHEET AND TOOLS

The following assessment worksheet and tools are used to work through the nursing process while engaged in a telephone interview. The worksheet includes a list of descriptors to help the nurse to remember to ask critical questions about patient symptoms. Space is devoted to notes on assessment, nursing diagnosis and problem solving, planning, and evaluation. A system review summary and whole-patient assessment tool are also provided. These tools can be copied and used near the phone to help the nurse to remember areas to be covered in the telephone interview.

Format: SOAP (Subjective, Objective, Assessment, Plan)

NURSING ASSESSMENT WORKSHEET

DESCRIPTORS (History of Present Illness — HPI)

1. Age, sex
2. Symptom onset
3. Location
4. Character
5. Radiation
6. Precipitating or aggravating factors
7. Relieving factors
8. Past treatment or evaluation and results
9. Course of symptom
10. Effect on normal activities
11. Associated Symptoms
12. Current Drugs or Medications

(PH) Significant past medical history:

ASSESSMENT
Subjective:

Objective:

NURSING DIAGNOSIS OR PROBLEM LIST
A:

PLAN
(Procedures; Common Medications; Patient Education, Referrals, Interventions, Outcomes):

EVALUATION
History, Assessment, Plan: What worked? What didn't? Why? What would you change? History? Problem diagnosis? Plan? How would you change it?

SYSTEM REVIEW SUMMARY

PSYCHOLOGICAL: Cognition, problem response, past response, cultural implications.

SOCIAL: Family relationships, occupational issues, economic status, patterns of care.

GENERAL: Weight change, fevers, fatigue, insomnia, swellings, temperature intolerance, back pain, skin disorder, smoking, alcohol, medications.

NP: Headaches, spells, dizziness, paresthesia, weakness, nervousness, depression, stroke.

EENT: Vision, hearing, tinnitus, frequent sore throats, sinus, dentures.

CVR: Chest pain, palpitations, dyspnea, orthopnea, cough, hemoptysis, hoarseness, wheeze, edema.

GI: Dysphagia, abdominal pain, indigestion, vomiting, constipation, diarrhea, melena, rectal blood, jaundice.

GU: Dysuria, frequency, nocturia, hematuria, stress incontinence, stream.

GYN: Interval, duration, amount, discomfort, leukorrhea, date of last menstrual period.

MS: Weakness, joint stiffness, muscle cramps, pain, swelling.

WHOLE PATIENT ASSESSMENT

The telephone nurse must listen accurately, and prioritize and organize information quickly and logically. This tool is designed to help the telephone nurse to remember areas for questioning during the assessment process. Copy it and place it near the phone for frequent reference.

Consider the characteristics of the patient and the risks concerning:

Age • Sex • General state • Anything which commands your attention

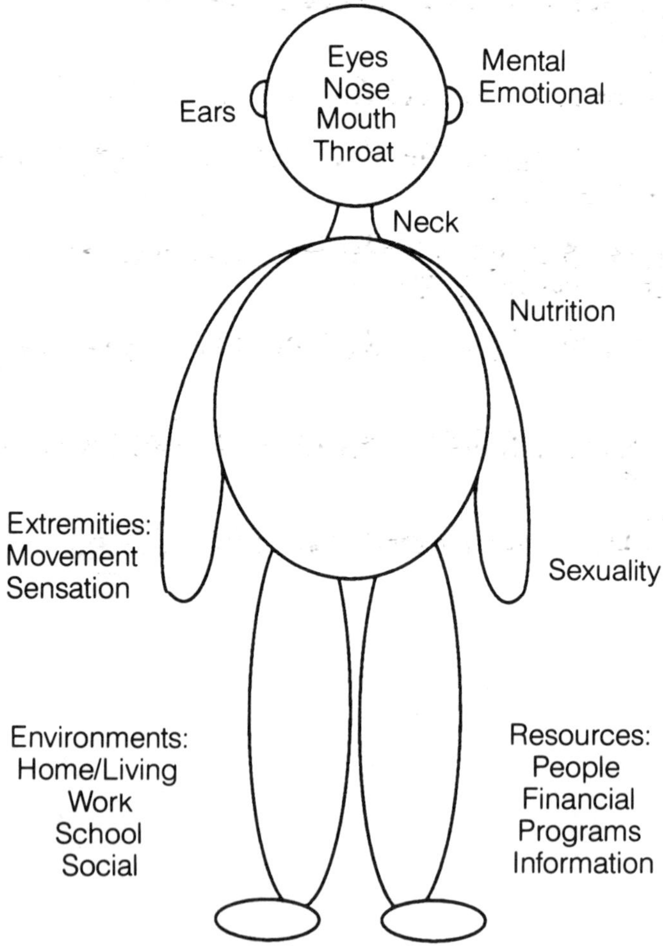

APPENDIX F

PEER EVALUATION FORM

Use this form to record your perceptions of the telephone nurse's success in achieving these important goals:

1. Adequately defines the nature and history of the caller's problems).

2. Adequately (and appropriately) explores caller's ideas, concerns, and expectations for the call.

3. Adequately (and appropriately) explores the effect that the problem(s) is having on the caller's activities of daily living.

4. Gives consideration to caller's risk factors: physical, psychosocial, environmental, etc.

5. Chooses appropriate recommendations/actions to deal with caller's problem(s).

6. Is able to communicate recommendations and actions effectively to the caller in such a way that the caller understands.

7. Is able to involve the caller in problem management.

8. Appropriately makes use of time, resources, referral sources, etc.

APPENDIX G

DISCUSSION EXERCISES

DISCUSSION EXERCISE #1

Mary Sue Young, 15, calls the Nurse on Call service. Mary Sue wants information about the organization's Formula Fast Diet, birth control, and what she can do about muscle aches and bruises. She doesn't want her parents to know about this call.

Clinical Considerations:

Professional, Ethical, and Legal Considerations:

How should the nurse proceed?
What questions should the nurse ask?

DISCUSSION EXERCISE #2

Donald Workman, 49 years old, is calling from his executive office. He had a routine complete physical exam and cardiac evaluation yesterday (ECG, treadmill, etc.). He is on his way out of town and is having some mild chest pains which go into his arms. His question: Can he take the muscle relaxant his physician gave him last year for a similar problem in his back?

Clinical Considerations:

Professional, Ethical, and Legal Considerations:

How should the nurse proceed?
What questions should the nurse ask?

DISCUSSION EXERCISE #3

An elderly sounding woman calls and refuses to give her name. She says she is having difficulty breathing and needs some help. She has a variety of medications and is alone in the house.

Clinical Considerations:

Professional, Ethical, and Legal Considerations:

How should the nurse proceed?
What questions should the nurse ask?

DISCUSSION EXERCISE #4

John Doe, age 24, calls and wants to know symptoms of AIDS.

Clinical Considerations:

Professional, Ethical, and Legal Considerations:

How should the nurse proceed?
What questions should the nurse ask?

APPENDIX H

THE NURSE ON CALL® PROGRAM

NURSE ON CALL is a turn-key telephone nursing program which provides organizations with everything they need to offer telephone nursing services to their constituents (patients, employees, industrial health clients, etc.).

HEALTHCARE ORGANIZATIONS

A number of benefits accrue to healthcare providers (hospitals, health maintenance organizations, physician clinics, etc.) offering NURSE ON CALL:

Improved Patient Access: Telephone nurses provide *timely and appropriate* healthcare information and advice to patients. The service provides a "one-stop shop" for caller's questions, allowing your organization to provide better, faster service to patients.

Improved Physician Support: NURSE ON CALL nurses can regularly communicate with physician's offices about their patients who have called the service; support physician on-call functions; offer physicians the opportunity to refer patients directly to NURSE ON CALL for nonurgent, after-hours questions; and provide a new form of "answering service" for physician practices.

Increased Revenue/Cut Costs: NURSE ON CALL helps the organization to control costs by facilitating the appropriate use of its medical resources. Referring callers to the appropriate level of care cuts waste and nonreimbursable costs. And because NURSE ON CALL engenders consumer goodwill, it can also assist in attracting new patients.

Improved Market Response/Visibility: As a new level of service for patients, NURSE ON CALL can position your organization as the most responsive to patient needs. In addition, it can increase the visibility of your organization and its services; assist your marketers in gathering market data; increase patient referrals to affiliated physicians, thereby increasing physician loyalty; and allow your organization to compete more effectively with other organizations offering alternative telephone-advice nursing systems.

EMPLOYERS

NURSE ON CALL is offered in a "Corporate Services" configuration, created specifically with the needs of employers in mind. The service, which is used in conjunction with existing benefits packages and/or employee assistance programs, offers professional telephone nursing services to assist employees in finding the right resources at the right time. These services, offered in other settings, have typically decreased inappropriate utilization, thereby lowering the cost of providing good care while improving satisfaction levels.

THE NURSE ON CALL PACKAGE

Included in the package is everything your organization needs to implement high-quality telephone nursing:

- NURSE ON CALL nursing guidelines software
- NURSE ON CALL patient tracking software
- NURSE ON CALL training program
- NURSE ON CALL telephone nursing guidelines (physician approved)
- NURSE ON CALL update
- clinical support services
- educational and marketing support services
- operations consulting

The package is further customized to fit the unique needs of your organization.

For more information, please contact:

Sandra C. Matherly
President
NURSE ON CALL
1007 Mapletree Lane
Mahomet, Illinois 61853
Tel. (217) 586-5558

REFERENCES

Abrams, William, and Robert Berko, editors. *The Merck Manual of Geriatrics.* Rahray, NJ: Merck, Sharp & Dohme Research Laboratories, 1990.

Alexander, Duane. "Women's Physical Health and Well Being." *Journal of the US Public Health Service*, Public Health Reports Supplement, July-August 1986, p. 10.

Alpern, B.B. *Reaching Women: The Way to Go in Marketing Healthcare Services*, Introduction, p.4. Chicago: Pluribus Press, 1987.

American Nurses' Association. "Nurses and Hospitals, Partners in Prevention" poster. 1989.

Banker, Burton, and Zieve, editors. *Principles of Ambulatory Medicine*. Baltimore, MD: Williams and Wilkins, 1986.

Benners and Tanner. "Clinical Judgment: How Expert Nurses Use Intuition." *American Journal of Nursing*, January 1987, p.23-31.

Botton, R. *People Skills*. Englewood Cliffs, NJ: Prentice-Hall, 1979.

Brown, J.L. *Telephone Medicine*. St. Louis: C. V. Mosby, 1980.

Brown, J. *Pediatric Telephone Medicine*. Philadelphia, PA: J.B. Lippincott, 1989.

Burton and Hazzard. "Geriatric Medicine: Special Considerations." *Principles of Ambulatory Medicine*, Chapter Six. Edited by Banker, Burton, and Zieve. Baltimore, MD: Williams and Wilkins, 1986.

Brume, Sheila. "Alcoholism and Women's Health." *Journal of the US Public Health Service*, Public Health Reports Supplement, July-August 1986, p. 38-41.

Chatham, Lois. "Issues Related to Alcohol, Drug Use and Abuse, and Mental Health of Women." *Journal of the US Public Health Service*, Public Health Reports Supplement, July-August 1986.

Curtin, Leah L. "Who or Why or Which or What?" editorial. *Nursing Management*, November 1984.

DiClemente, R.J. "Minorities and AIDS: Knowledge, Attitudes, and Misconceptions Among Black and Latino Adolescents." American Journal of Public Health, January 1988, p.55.

Dreyfus, H.S. *Mind Over Machine: The Power of Human Intuition and Expertise in the Era of the Computer*. New York: Free Press, 1985.

Edelman and Mendel. *Health Promotion Throughout the Lifespan*, "Infancy." St. Louis: C.V. Mosby, 1986.

Fish, R., and M. Ehrhardt. *Malpractice: Managing Your Defense*. Oradell, NJ: Medical Economics, 1986.

Gallegher and Kreidler. *Nursing and Health: Maximizing Human Potential Throughout the Lifecycle*, "Maximizing the Health of the Infant." East Norwalk, CT: Appleton and Lange, 1987.

Gentry, J.H.H. "Social Factors Affecting Women's Health." *Journal of the Public Health Service*, Public Health Reports Supplement, July-August 1986.

Group Health Cooperative of Puget Sound. *Nurses Guide to Telephone Triage and Health Care*. Baltimore: Williams and Wilkins, 1986.

Gordon, Marjorie. *Manual of Nursing Diagnosis*. New York: McGraw-Hill, 1982.

Gordon, Marjorie. *Nursing Diagnosis: Process and Application*. New York: McGraw-Hill, 1982.

Johnson, T.M. et al. Letter to editor. *Journal of the American Association*, March 7, 1986.

Julty. *Men's Bodies, Men's Selves*. New York, NY: Dell, 1979.

Kane, Ouslander, and Abrass. *Essentials of Clinical Geriatrics*. New York: McGraw-Hill, 1989.

Knutson, D'Angelo, DesChamps, Steiner, Matherly, and Rochester. *Ambulatory Care Nursing Standards and Performance Evaluations*. Denver, CO: Center for Research in Ambulatory Health Care Administration, 1987.

Kolb, L. *Modern Clinical Psychiatry*. Philadelphia: Saunders, 1982.

Leninger, Madeleine. "Transcultural Care Diversity and Universality: A Theory of Nursing." *Nursing and Healthcare*, April 1985.

Magill, Williams, and Caspi. "Patient Education: Progress and Problems." *Nursing Management*, February 1986.

Malasanos, Barkauskas, Moss, and Allen. *Health Assessment*, 4th ed. St. Louis: C.V. Mosby, 1990.

Mancini, M., and A. Gale. *Emergency Care and the Law*. Rockville, MD: Aspen Publications, 1987.

Martinelli, A.M. "Pain and Ethnicity: How People of Different Cultures Experience Pain." *Association of Operating Room Nurses Journal*, August 1987.

McDonough, William J. "Risk Management Briefs." *Journal of Medical Practice Management*, Winter 1990.

McGear and Simms. *Telephone Triage and Management*. Philadelphia, PA: Saunders, 1988.

Moore and Dworkin. "Ethnographic Methodologic Assessment of Pain Perceptions by Verbal Description." *Pain*, 1988, p.195-204.

Murchison, I., et al. *Legal Accountability in the Nursing Process*. St. Louis: C.V. Mosby, 1978.

Murray and Zentner. *Nursing Assessment and Health Promotion Strategies Throughout the Life Span*, 4th ed. East Norwalk, CT: Appleton & Lange, 1989.

Pagana, Kathleen, and Timothy Pagana. *Pocket Nurse Guide to Physical Assessment*. St. Louis: C.V. Mosby, 1986.

Potter, Patricia. *Pocket Nurse Guide to Physical Assessment*. St. Louis: C.V. Mosby, 1986.

Rosekrans, Julia, et al. *Pediatric Telephone Guidelines*. Darien, CT: Patient Care Publications, 1979.

Rosenbaum, J.N. "Depression: Viewed from a Transcultural Nursing Theoretical Perspective." *Journal of Advanced Nursing*, 1989, p.14.

Schaefer, M.S. "To Avoid a Lawsuit, Keep the Record Straight." *RN*, November 1981, p.81-84.

Schlotfeldt, Rozella. "This I Believe...Nursing is Health Care." *Nursing Outlook*, April 1972, p.245-246.

Sherman and Fields. *Guide to Patient Evaluation*. New York, NY: Medical Examination Publishing Co., 1974.

Smith, Carol E. "With Good Assessment Skills, You Can Construct a Solid Framework for Patient Care." *Nursing 84*, December 1984.

Statistical Abstract of the United States, 1989.

Thayer, M.B. "Telephone Management." *Pediatric Nursing*, March/April 1984, p.121-122+.

Tubesing, Donald. *Kicking Your Stress Habits*. Duluth, MN: Whole Person Associates, 1981.

Tucker, Susan Martin, et al. *Patient Care Standards*. St. Louis: C.V. Mosby, 1984.

Von Oech. *A Whack on the Side of the Head*. Berkeley, CA: Ten Speed Press, 1985.

Wasson, John, et al. *The Common Symptom Guide*, 2nd ed. New York: McGraw-Hill, 1984.

Weed, L.L. *Medical Records, Medical Education and Patient Care*. Chicago: Yearbook Medical Publishers, 1970.

Weisman, Carol S. "Communication Between Women and Their Healthcare Providers: Research Findings and Unanswered Questions." *Journal of the US Public Health Service*, Public Health Reports Supplement, July-August 1986, p.147.

White, Peggi. "Client Perception of the Quality of Advice by the Registered Nurses in a Telephone Nursing Service." Master's thesis, University of Illinois, Chicago, 1989.

Whitten and Cameron. *Developing Management Skills*. Glenview, IL: Scott, Foresman and Co., 1984.

Zander, Karen. *Primary Nursing*. Rockville, MD: Aspen Publications, 1980.